LOSE LICENSE LOSE FREEDOM

Essential Information for Aging Baby Boomers Who Want to Keep their License and Continue to Enjoy the Open Road

by Michael Vaughan

Copyright © 2014 by Michael Vaughan
First Edition – July 2014

ISBN
978-1-4602-4869-0 (Hardcover)
978-1-4602-4870-6 (Paperback)
978-1-4602-4871-3 (eBook)

All rights reserved.

No part of this publication may be reproduced in any form, or by any means, electronic or mechanical, including photocopying, recording, or any information browsing, storage, or retrieval system, without permission in writing from the publisher.

Produced by:

FriesenPress
Suite 300 – 852 Fort Street
Victoria, BC, Canada V8W 1H8

www.friesenpress.com

Distributed to the trade by The Ingram Book Company

TABLE OF CONTENTS

CHAPTER 1
What's the Problem?..1

CHAPTER 2
Your Clock is Running..12

CHAPTER 3
The People Who Can Take Your License Away............28

CHAPTER 4
Pass the Test..42

CHAPTER 5
Who's in Charge Here?
The Data or the Driver?..58

CHAPTER 6
New Technology for Accident Free Driving................70

CHAPTER 7
My Top Fifty Picks..92

CHAPTER 8
Road Trips to Remember..146

CHAPTER 9
DRIVE ON!..184

ABOUT THE AUTHOR

CHAPTER 1

What's the Problem?

George Weller

On July 16, 2003, George Weller, age 86, ploughed through two and a half blocks of the Santa Monica, California farmer's market at speeds between 40 and 60 mph (60 and 100 km/h).

Witnesses testified that he was staring straight ahead with both hands on the steering wheel while bodies flew over the hood of his car as he yelled, "Get out of the way." Weller killed 10 people and seriously injured 63 others.

Shortly afterwards, video surfaced of a previous accident Weller had been in ten years earlier. It showed Weller had driven his car off the road, just like in the farmer's market accident, and was wandering in a confused state around his crashed car, in a populated, public area.

After the Santa Monica episode, Weller was eventually found guilty of 10 counts of vehicular manslaughter but never went to jail. By the time of his conviction, he was nearly 90 years old and suffering from heart disease. The judge decided that putting Weller in jail would just be a burden to taxpayers.

The tragedy caused by Weller was the worst of its kind though there have been many similar but less deadly cases. Ten years after Weller, 100-year-old Preston Carter backed his car out of a parking lot in Los Angeles and onto a sidewalk across from an elementary school. He hit 14 people, including 11 children.

The screams didn't cause him to stop nor did the people who pounded on his windows. "He was not paying attention," said a witness.

Police confirmed that Carter had a valid driver's license and insurance.

It shows that a decade after Weller killed 10 people, governments still haven't come up with an effective way to handle the problem of aging drivers.

Spend Five Minutes on Google

Go to Google News and just type in "elderly driver." Here's what you'll get – an endless string of stories like these:

"An elderly driver accidentally crashed her pickup truck into a Las Vegas grocery store on Saturday, injuring 26 people and sending 9 to the hospital, police said. It was unclear why the woman, who was in her mid-80s, drove into the Food 4 Less store but it did not appear to be deliberate."

"An elderly couple is recovering in hospital after crashing their car into a Vancouver apartment complex Wednesday afternoon. The driver, a man believed to be in his mid-80s, lost control of the vehicle while coming down a driveway and hit a concrete wall. The vehicle then flipped over and came to a rest beside the building's pool."

"An elderly woman crashed her silver Ford Focus into a Laval, Quebec daycare centre. Three children were immediately rushed to hospital for treatment, along with the 80-year-old driver of the car."

Public Opinion is Against You

It's becoming conventional wisdom that all older drivers are a menace on the road and must be removed. But people don't all age in the same way. There are lots of 80-year-olds who go skiing and do push-ups while others, who are much younger, can barely move – or think.

Banning everyone over a certain age from driving would be arbitrary and unreasonable and as a result is rarely ever done. Instead we get piecemeal efforts on a state-by-state or province-by-province basis. Unsafe drivers by the thousands remain on the road while people who are fully capable of driving have their licenses pulled or get shamed into handing over their keys.

The problem will get much worse as Baby Boomers hit their retirement years by the millions. By 2050, almost 1 in 4 people will be over 65 and 1 in 10 will be over 80. Everyone seems to recognize the issue but governments aren't prepared to deal with it.

We should be evaluating older drivers on the basis of their motor skills and cognitive abilities and not their date of birth. Some jurisdictions require additional screening for license renewal after someone hits a certain age but the testing, in many cases, is a joke. Comprehensive testing is thought to be too expensive or difficult to administer but believe me, it is coming.

The aging process is different for everyone. When the screening tools arrive, they should be function-based rather than age-based. There is a huge multi-year, multi-million dollar study from Transport Canada and others that is developing better ways of identifying older drivers who are truly at risk. We'll get to that in a lot more detail in Chapter 3.

How Dangerous Are You?

The myth that older drivers are more accident prone than other motorists is just that—a myth, according to a new study by the Insurance Institute for Highway Safety (IIHS). That's the insurance industry's research organization and their report shows crashes involving older Americans have declined during the past 15 years.

The rate of fatal crashes among drivers age 70 and older fell 42% per licensed driver between 1997 and 2012, outpacing the 30% drop for drivers aged 35 to 54 over the same period. That's good news because the aging Baby Boom generation is putting more and more elderly drivers on the roads. The number of licensed drivers older than 70 increased 30% between 1997 and 2012 and that will continue.

The report states, "It's a marked shift that began to take hold in the mid-1990s and indicates that the growing ranks of aging drivers aren't making U.S. roads deadlier."

Older drivers have lower police-reported crash rates per person than younger drivers, largely because they drive less.

"Older drivers are not only less likely to crash in recent years; they also are sharing in the benefits of newer and safer vehicles. It also helps that older people in general are more fit than in years past," said Anne McCartt, IIHS's senior vice-president for research and a coauthor of the study.

Seniors as a group may be pretty much as safe as anyone else on the road but other studies have shown that when they are in an accident they come out worse than younger drivers. An accident that can leave a 20-year-old with a bump on the knee can mean broken bones and a hospital admission to someone much older. And of course, the elderly are more at risk of injury as pedestrians than they are as drivers.

At the Crossroads

Most older drivers are good at recognising age-related changes and they adjust their driving accordingly. This is "self-regulation" and it will be explored in detail a little later on.

But something interesting a US study found was that 37% of fatalities and 60% of injuries experienced by older drivers take place at intersections. A British study found similar results, along with a large number of accidents for older drivers merging into the traffic on motorways. An ordinary right turn is difficult for older drivers, said the study by the British Automobile Association, "...because roads have become so much busier they are forced to take risks at an age when it is harder to judge the speed of approaching vehicles."

Because the Brits drive on the left side of the road, the right turns over there are the equivalent of left turns in North America - and, yes, it's the left turns that cause the most problems for North American elderly drivers.

This is pointing out that there's a problem with an unknown number of drivers with cognitive impairment, who can't or won't recognise age-related changes. Those are the ones we should be targeting and the "science" exists to do just that.

Who's Still Driving?

Nearly everyone. Seniors realize that if they lose their licenses, there's a high probability they'll become shut-ins.

In 2009, Statistics Canada did a big survey and discovered, "3.25 million people aged 65 and over have a driver's license—three-quarters of all Seniors. Of that number, about 200,000 are aged 85 and over. Of all those over 85 who are licensed; 67% are men and 26% are women. Since people in their 80s and over are, and will continue to be, a fast-growing segment of the Senior population, the number of elderly drivers will also continue to increase at a rapid pace."

The last thing a Senior wants is to be trapped in his or her own home. Statscan reported, "A majority of Seniors live in areas where the car is the primary form of transportation. Thus, it is not surprising to find that the majority of Seniors, even those of more advanced ages, travel mostly by car. The majority of Seniors have no intention of moving and plan to remain where they live as long as possible."

Statscan also discovered that even having poor eyesight or cognitive problems does not always mean an end to driving.

"A majority of Seniors have adequate visual, cognitive, and auditory functions and most Seniors drive their cars to get around. However, some 14,000 Seniors who have very limited sight (they are unable to read the newspaper or recognize a friend on the other side of the street, even with glasses) still have a license."

That is also the case for 40,000 Seniors who had a driver's license but were very likely to forget things and had considerable difficulty thinking clearly and solving everyday problems. In addition, about 20,000 people who had been diagnosed with Alzheimer's disease or some other form of dementia had a driver's license.

Seniors appear to be determined to hang onto their licenses just as long as is humanly possible and seem to have little use for public transit. "Among men aged 65 to 74, 84% get around mainly by driving their cars, and 9% by being passengers in cars. That leaves 4% using public transit, 3% walking or bicycling, and the rest using accessible transit or taxis."

HOMEWORK ASSIGNMENT

Go to the computer. Punch up YouTube and enter 23½ *Hours* in the Search window.

You're going to be hearing from Dr. Mike Evans in a brilliant little eight-minute video now. Doc Evans is going to explain to you the entry requirements for continued safe driving.

If you don't buy into his message, you have wasted your money on this book – and sorry, no refunds are available. So check out 23½ *Hours* now and we'll talk later.

Dr. Mike Evans wrote and narrated that video. Including you and me, it has now been viewed by about nine million people. I buy into his views about the health benefits of exercise one hundred %.

Is Self-Regulation Enough?

Age alone does not make a bad driver. Vision, hearing and other physical abilities decline with age but if you stay in shape, it could take a very long time until your driving skills reach the point where your license should be taken away.

Being stripped of a license simply for reaching a certain age may happen eventually - though probably not while enough Boomers are around as active voters. But the introduction of tough older-driver testing is inevitable.

At the present time in many jurisdictions, you have to re-apply for your driving license at the age of 70 and every so often thereafter. At this point very, very few jurisdictions require a medical exam or a driving test. Count on both of those things being required soon.

Until then, you have the ultimate responsibility for deciding whether you're fit or unfit for driving. This is "self-regulation."

The prevailing wisdom seems to be that those who wish to continue driving beyond, say, the age of 70 should only be prevented from doing so if there are compelling reasons.

One reason for this tolerant attitude is the fact that the roads have become safer and safer for everyone over the past 40 years. That has been the result of a combination of things; safer car design, seatbelt laws, a crackdown on drunk driving, and the introduction of graduated licensing for teens.

Teens still pose the greatest risk on the road and crash more often than any other age group, including 80-year-olds.

Many older drivers self-regulate by driving less and refraining from driving at night. But of course not all older drivers are that responsible. At least teenage drivers are subjected to a tough testing process and generally only gain driving rights in gradual stages. Older drivers should see the writing on the wall.

What's holding back these stricter regulations? Cost for one thing; road-testing older drivers is expensive. But there's politics too. Older people vote and they know how to vote their interests as a demographic group. Plus their voter turnout is much higher than the Gen Y crowd's.

So, the Baby Boomer, who's had the best of the Golden Age of inexpensive, unregulated driving, is still in control today. But as an old geezer named Bob Dylan, who I recently saw on TV peddling Dodges, once said, "The times they are a-changin.'"

You Will be Judged…by a Younger Car-Hating Generation

According to the Federal Highway Administration, only 46% of potential drivers 19 years old and younger had driver's licenses in 2008 – down from 64% just a decade earlier. Go into an auto dealership and it will probably look like a Senior Center.

The car-loving Baby Boomers are going to get little sympathy from the younger generations, who will be setting the rules about who is fit to drive. There is a major cultural and political shift taking place, when it comes to car ownership and enjoyment.

I recently asked a 20-something-year-old, "What do you like least about your city?" She answered instantly, "Driving in it." Young people are turning away in droves from what was once the dream and the status of car ownership.

Today the cost of cars and fuel, the insurance, the permits, the radar cops in revenue traps, the lack of parking, and the gridlock everywhere is turning kids against our former freedom machines.

And guess who is going to set the rules that will get "all those dangerous old people off the road?" Not you or me. It'll be the Millennials.

Tough, tough regulations are coming. If you want to stay in the game – prepare now.

The purpose of this book, as I have stated, is not to argue that drivers who are a danger to themselves or others should remain on the road.

This book is for the Boomers who decide to stay healthy, who sharpen their driving skills, and who understand and use new safety technology. You have to get ready to deal with the licensing and insurance realities that are looming. If you don't, by the time you hit 70, your days of transportation freedom will be over forever.

The Boomer generation that's heading towards retirement now is better educated and healthier than any generation before it. That makes Boomers worthy opponents in the potential war of generations, over how to pay for the rising social welfare costs of an increasingly older society, and over who is fit to drive.

FEATURE INTERVIEW

To get a little deeper into this question of the mysterious Millennials, let's have a chat now with Jim Farley; Executive Vice-President of Global Marketing, Ford Motor Company. Jim is in charge of all the research, marketing, and communications at Ford and he is also the head of Lincoln; Ford's luxury division.

Vaughan

Is the lack of interest in driving among Millennials going to kill the car business?

Farley

This is interesting because working on various projects, I've been able to track this. It's the largest cohort of customers our industry has seen and usually those cohorts have different brand preferences, different upper body silhouette preferences and they change our industry. So I think they will have as big an impact, if not more, on our industry than their parents, the Boomers.

Vaughan

But they're not getting drivers' licenses. There's plenty of research on that.

Farley

That's true. But when I look below the surface, what I see is something that's a little different from what our industry dialogue is. First of all, getting a license now is very expensive. It's not part of the free curriculum like it used to be in high school. It was so easy for us to get our licenses – that's not the case anymore. And people are busy. But what we are seeing is that as Millennials start to form families, they are buying vehicles as fast as their parents. So I think when we see that large group of Millennials start to form families, we will really learn whether they are car shoppers or not. Independent transportation – even with the great public transportation choices now – is still really appealing. I think it's going to take a little more time because they're under a lot more pressure. I'm very hopeful. I also think they'll change our industry in a fundamental way.

Vaughan

So if I read you right, the automotive industry has finally taken its focus off the Boomers. Boomers are now officially yesterday.

Farley

No, I don't mean that at all. The Boomers are actually the core customers in our industry, in the Americas and Europe. When you look at China though, the average buyer in China is at least fifteen to twenty years younger. So the China market now being the largest market in the world – absolutely that's a Millennial market. But they think much differently than the Millennials in the Western world.

The Boomers will continue to drive the market and they're going to look for more as they go into retirement. They're going to look for more specialty cars. They're going to want space. They're going to want stuff that's more for them. Some will downsize to simplify their lives. Some with more money will buy more fancy specialty cars. So we could see a whole resurgence of specialty cars like Mustang. But their kids – they are really different. The jury is still out awbout how many of them will be car buyers.

And I'm still very hopeful but their preferences will be different. For example – will they buy an Odyssey or a Sienna or will they turn to a Transit Connect wagon? What we have seen over the last thirty or forty years in Canada and in the U.S. is that when people go into the family-forming life stage, they tend to not buy what their parents bought. The station wagons turn into minivans. Minivans turn into SUVs. I am absolutely convinced that this wave of Millennials will pick body styles that will surprise all of us and that will be different than their parents.

. . . .

CHAPTER 2

Your Clock is Running

Over the years, brains and bodies change – and not for the better.

By 2025, people aged 65 and older will account for 25% of Canadian and US drivers. That's a lot of people who have lost a lot of skill.

Here's the safety and mobility crisis that looms for aging Baby Boomers and their families. Somehow they (or the authorities) have to determine:

1. Whether they remain capable of safely operating a motor vehicle. If not:
2. Can their driving skills be improved to the point where they can remain on the road? If not:
3. How they can continue to be mobile?

Let's take a look at the skills that decline and see if managing these changes will extend your safe driving years.

Motor Skills

Driving a car is a physical activity as well as a mental activity. To drive safely, you need a certain amount of physical strength, flexibility, and coordination. Taken together, these abilities define your motor skills.

Strength isn't as much of an issue as it used to be, way back before power steering, power brakes, power windows, power seats etc. etc., became standard on nearly every car.

Flexibility decreases as you get older. Proper exercise will improve your flexibility and you'll need it if you get re-tested. You'll have to show you can reach for and buckle your safety belt, turn to check blind spots, and grip and control the steering wheel.

You'll have to have enough coordination to use the foot pedals, adjust mirrors to minimize blind spots, and operate other controls for headlights, windshield wipers, and so on.

Vision Issues

None of your senses is more important to safe driving than vision. Nearly all the sensory input you need to drive a car comes from visual cues. If your eyesight is seriously diminished, your ability to drive safely falls off a cliff - an apt metaphor if there ever was one.

It's only logical that most provinces and states require motorists to undergo vision tests as part of the driver's license renewal process. It depends on where you live - you may have your vision tested at a licensing office or by a private optometrist.

Tunnel Vision

Another issue is that as you age, your useful field of view gets smaller. Peripheral vision problems mean that you don't have a normal, wide-angle field of vision, even though your central vision may be fine. As it gets worse, it causes the sensation of seeing through a narrow tube, or "tunnel vision."

A common cause of loss of peripheral vision is optic-nerve damage from glaucoma. If tunnel vision comes on suddenly, see your eye doctor immediately. It may indicate a detached retina, which is a medical emergency that must be treated as soon as possible to avoid permanent vision loss.

Unfortunately, eyeglasses or contact lenses will not correct permanent loss of peripheral vision.

Sharpness of Vision & Changing Focus

Here's a driver licensing standard that varies widely across North America – it's called best-corrected visual acuity, or best distance vision with eyeglasses or contact lenses.

We all know that if we have good eyesight (normal visual acuity), we have 20/20 vision.

Over the years, eye doctors have decided what a normal person should be able to see when standing 20 feet away from an eye chart. If you have 20/20 vision, it means you can see what all the other so-called normal people can see.

But if you have 20/40 vision, it means that when you stand 20 feet away from the chart you can see what a normal person can see when standing 40 feet from the chart.

20/100 means that when you stand 20 feet from the chart, you can see what a normal person sees standing 100 feet away. 20/200 is generally the definition of legal blindness.

If you have trouble with your vision, you need to get tested for nearsightedness (myopia) and/or farsightedness (hyperopia) and yes, you can have both.

Nearsighted people have difficulty seeing objects at a distance, but are fine reading a book. Nearsightedness can be corrected with glasses, contact lenses, or eye surgery. Some people with nearsightedness may need to wear glasses or contact lenses all the time, or only for distance vision; such as when driving.

Hyperopia, or farsightedness, is a common vision problem. People with farsightedness can see distant objects very well, but have difficulty focusing on objects that are close.

However, even if your vision tests well in an office, your vision can still be effectively reduced on the road at night.

Night Vision

By the age 60, your eyes could need three times as much light to see as they did at age 20.

That's because over the years, the muscles that control pupil size, in reaction to light, lose some strength. This causes the pupil to become smaller and widen (dilate) less in dark conditions, making it harder to see.

The result is that a driver aged-60 not only may need three times as much light to see as a teenager, it may also take more than twice as long to adjust to a change from light to darkness.

Poor night vision makes night driving hazardous, especially when the ability to see through glare also decreases with age.

Driving at night adds degrees of difficulty for all drivers, but Seniors face increased risk because of the factors discussed above. These are the reasons why many older adults limit or regulate their driving. Many Seniors decide to drive only during the day.

If you cannot avoid driving at night, slow down, keep your eyes moving, and protect your eyes from glare. If you get blinded by oncoming high beams, look down toward the right side of the road and keep your eyes on the painted line until the vehicle passes. But a better idea is to simply skip the night driving.

Hearing

Hearing loss is one of the most common conditions affecting older adults. It starts to set into people after age 50 and by the time they're 65, about one-third of people have it; especially men.

Safety problems occur around traffic if you can't hear horns, or sirens, or railway crossing bells. Hearing loss can often be corrected with hearing aids although many people who need them avoid them out of personal vanity.

Slower Reaction Time

When you're driving a car you're making decisions constantly; you have to be able to pull in information from several sources at once and make split-second decisions. This happens automatically when you're younger but the reaction time can and will slow down as you age. Slow reaction time can put you in some dangerous situations.

Pain or stiffness in muscles or joints can also slow you down when you're trying to react quickly in an emergency.

The best way to improve reaction time is to exercise your mind and body. Go back to Chapter 1 and the Doc Evans program for the best advice on the physical exercise issue. As for keeping "the little grey cells" working – in the following pages, you're going to see some actual tests that government-recognized driving assessment programs use.

What to do About It

So let's assume your information-processing speed is tailing off slightly and your eyesight, while still legal, isn't what it was. There are ways to compensate.

Let's deal with the big issue first and that would be distracted driving. We all know from the statistics that distracted driving is as dangerous as drunk driving.

The Ontario government states that distracted driving is cited as a causal factor in 30% to 50% of traffic collisions in the province but it may be higher, due to under-reporting.

So, especially as you get older, you must eliminate distractions inside the vehicle. The big one – now illegal in any intelligent jurisdiction – is talking or texting on a handheld device. Still, I would wager that every day all of you who drive will see other drivers texting and talking while paying lots of attention to their handheld devices. I was nearly run off the road on a four-lane highway recently, by a woman in a big SUV who was texting away while almost pushing me off the shoulder.

There has been an increase in pedestrian fatalities in North America, after a five-year decline, and I think it is certain to have something to do with the explosion of texting on cell phones. So that's definitely out – but what else is defined as distracted driving?

Whose Definition of Distracted Driving?

As a little experiment, an insurance company sent a bunch of spotters out on the highways and byways to identify distracted drivers. The spotters bagged 1400 of them and issued a press release on their catch.

Guess what? The most common offence documented was eating or drinking. The survey identified 25% of all distracted perpetrators as consuming food or beverages.

Talking to passengers was the second most reported infraction, and smoking while driving was next. Why do they put cup-holders in cars if you aren't to be allowed to sip a coffee while on the road? Smoking is obviously terrible for your health but should it be reported as a distracted driving offence?

Is talking to a passenger a danger on our roads? I'm not sure about that one. But according to observers, talking on a handheld device and/or texting finished at a distant 15%.

To repeat, I am all in favour of enforcing laws against driving while texting, as much as I am for the laws against driving while impaired. I personally think "consuming food or beverages" shouldn't be a crime – but times are changing.

In Illinois, there's a municipal movement that's trying to get any form of eating while driving declared an offence. I don't think that's reasonable. A sandwich, or shall we say a donut for you law enforcement officials, is easily managed. If you're using a knife and fork, then you should probably be booked.

Nevertheless, as we get older we have to take a very serious view of these things. Even reaching over to adjust the radio volume can take your eyes off the road for a second and can you really afford it? You need to keep the environment inside your vehicle calm and distraction-free.

Distracted Driving in Aircraft?

Distracted driving isn't only a serious issue on the road; now unfortunately, it appears to be in the air as well. An investigation by the U.S. National Transportation Safety Board (NTSB) found that text messages were a contributing factor in the crash of a medical air-ambulance helicopter that crashed in Missouri in 2011, killing all four people on board. Investigators concluded that the pilot was distracted by personal text messages before and during the fatal flight. The NTSB has since recommended banning the use of portable electronic devices by all flight-crew members.

Phone Addiction

I read an interesting article online, not too long ago, in *Medical Daily* titled, "Warning Signs of a Cell Phone Addict." There's a psychological term now to describe people who obsessively check for emails and messages – it's called "nomophobia" an abbreviation of no mobile phone phobia, which of course is the fear of being without a mobile phone.

A psychotherapist quoted in the article says cell phones are as addictive as slot machines and cause people to become disengaged from having face-to-face relationships.

"The lives of cell phone addicts are so contingent on their need to feel socially connected on their phones that without mobile technology, they begin to express a sense of vulnerability that can trigger certain moods and behaviours," wrote reporter Lizette Borreli.

I witness the excessive compulsion to check a mobile phone every day. I do not carry one personally but all around me, I see people who constantly take their phones from their pockets and nervously start pressing buttons…often it's the driver in the car next to me.

Whether cell phone usage is an addiction or an obsessive-compulsive disorder I can't say but as a cause of traffic accidents and fatalities, it is a major problem. Older people have the advantage of not having grown up with smart phones in their cradles and should be less likely to fall into "nomophobia."

War on Texting

Governor Andrew Cuomo of New York, a savvy politician if there was ever one, is on the issue. Cuomo has announced, "New York State is continuing to use every tool at its disposal to combat texting while driving."

He has decided to set up special texting zones on the side of state highways and the thruway, to allow motorists to pull over and use their phones. There will be 91 of them for starters, using existing rest areas and service centres as a way to encourage drivers to get off the road before using their cell phones.

It's hard to battle an addiction but this seems like a sensible idea. The "texting zone" announcement is part of a big campaign by Cuomo's government to fight cell phone use by drivers. They have more unmarked police cars hunting for offenders and Cuomo proudly announced that troopers gave out 21,580 tickets in a recent summer – a 365% increase over the previous year.

HOMEWORK ASSIGNMENT

Get back on YouTube

There is a short film you do not want to miss from from Werner Herzog. It's a 35- minute online documentary titled, *From One Second to the Next*. It describes in horrifying detail, four accidents caused when a driver was texting behind the wheel. The film was commissioned by AT&T to be shown to high schools, safety groups, and government agencies across the U.S. – it is definitely worth viewing. So get on YouTube and type in *From One Second to the Next*.

Is Voice-to-Text Technology Any Better?

A number of automakers have been adding supposedly safer voice-to-text features to their vehicles and I have tried out many of them.

Sometimes, the voice recognition system works fine, if you tell it turn up the heat or change the radio station but plenty of times, it doesn't. It shouts back at you, "Invalid Command" or some such phrase and tells you to try again. Sometimes it will list a bunch of "valid" commands and tell you to choose one. Some systems display the valid commands and you take your eyes off the road to read them. Most of the time, I yell back at the damned system or start pushing buttons on the touch screen; in either case, I'm seriously distracted.

Well now there's a new study by the Texas Transportation Institute, which warns that this hands-free voice recognition technology is likely to leave drivers distracted and at risk of a crash as much as monkeying with their cell phones. Despite it being billed as a safer alternative, the new study indicates that texting in any form, including voice-operated texting, is a dangerous distraction.

The study took 43 licensed drivers between the ages of 16 and 60 and sent them driving on a closed course, four times. They were asked to drive once while focusing on the road, once while texting manually, once using an iPhone voice-to-text app, and once using an Android one.

"Results indicate that driver reaction times were nearly two times slower than the baseline condition, no matter which texting method was used," according to Christine Yager of the Texas Transportation Institute. It's interesting to note that the drivers perceived the voice-operated systems to be safer but the study showed driving performance suffered equally. In fact, in some cases, manual texting actually took less time to complete.

As I have discovered, voice-to-text technology isn't perfect and when you start arguing with the thing, you are taking your concentration off the road. The National Transportation Safety Board has outlined an aggressive plan to eliminate most high-tech distractions from the automobile, including not just Bluetooth systems but even most onboard navigation devices.

The battle over the safety of voice-based systems is just getting started.

Pets in Cars Increase Crash Rates

Researchers at the University of Alabama, Birmingham claim that Seniors who drive with pets in the car are twice as likely to end up in a crash. "This is the first study to evaluate the presence of pets in a vehicle as a potential internal distraction for elderly drivers," said Gerald McGwin, Ph.D., the senior author of the study.

According to NHTSA, drivers should never take their eyes off the road for more than two seconds at a time. A moving pet, especially in the front seat, can cause a driver to do exactly that. A couple of days ago I saw a woman barrelling down our street with a small dog in her lap with its head stuck out the window. Oftentimes I see a large dog sitting in the front passenger seat beside a Senior.

I think an animal loose in the front seat should automatically result in the driver getting a distracted driving fine. If a dog or cat gets startled and moves suddenly it stands a very good chance of causing the driver to lose control of the vehicle. "Adding another distracting element, especially an active, potentially moving animal, provides more opportunity for an older driver to respond to a driving situation in a less than satisfactory way," said Prof. McGwin.

Distracting Signage

Roadside billboards are a form of advertising that you can't turn off. They're also a cause of distracted driving. And don't get me started on those Jumbotrons along the side of expressways! These digital billboards are huge, energy- wasting, outdoor TV screens – they are there to deliberately make you watch television instead of watching the road. I would have them banned immediately.

According to the California Department of Motor Vehicles, 80% of crashes and 65% of near-crashes involve driver distraction within 3 seconds of the crash and the department classifies looking at billboards as a distraction. In other words, ignore these ugly outdoor TV screens and any other form of advertising that takes your attention away from the task at hand.

File Your Flight Plan

If you are a private pilot travelling more than 25 nautical miles from your point of departure, you must file either a flight plan or a flight itinerary. It would include information about your aircraft, your route, and the time your trip will take. If you don't show up and close your flight plan within an hour of your filed arrival time, you are considered overdue and a search begins.

When you're driving your car you don't have any an air traffic controllers or flight service specialists to deal with but a Drive Plan for the older driver makes a lot of sense.

Plan your route before you get behind the wheel.

First of all, thinking your journey through means you avoid having to make last-minute decisions about where to turn or how to find your destination.

If high-speed highways and major roads with heavy traffic stress you out – avoid them. Use local roads instead of highways and steer clear of rush hours.

Estimate your time of arrival conservatively so you won't feel you're running late every time you look at the clock. You're not in a race – take your time.

Increase your following distance. Allow a greater distance between you and the vehicle ahead of you, so you'll have more time to slow down or stop.

In the city, you may want to minimize left turns. Older drivers get more than their share of accidents in crashes involving left-hand turns. You may want to plan to make three right turns in place of a difficult left. Or maybe only turn left in intersections with designated left-hand turn lanes.

Review your meds. Prescription and over-the-counter medications can slow your reflexes and make you sleepy. Drowsy driving is as dangerous as drunk driving. Be sure to get enough sleep before a long trip and take lots of breaks along the way.

Later on, we're going to get into the matter of selecting a vehicle with Senior-friendly features and even driver assistance technologies – but now let's see how one of the major automakers is thinking about older drivers.

FEATURE INTERVIEW

With Sheryl Connelly, Manager of Global Trends and Futuring, Ford Motor Company

Her title means that Sheryl Connelly is Ford's Futurist; her job to predict new trends at least 3 years in advance. She's also the only person from the automotive industry named to *Fast Company*'s Top 100 Most Creative People in Business for 2013. Connelly is up to speed on Ford safety technologies like reverse sensing systems, camera rear vision, adaptive cruise control and the blind spot alert and she insists they're not just for the older demographic. I couldn't agree more. Advanced safety helps everyone.

Vaughan

It's all about Boomers. In ten years, 25% of the drivers on the road will be 65 or over.

Connelly

The aging population is one of the biggest trends worldwide and the Baby Boomers are a big part of it. The Boomers created the middle class. They were the organizational men. They worked really hard and were very concerned about the financial security of their families. They liked big homes and expensive cars. Now they're getting to new life stage.

Vaughan

Ten thousand a day are now reaching age 65.

Connelly

Baby boomers have been really proactive and vital to retain their health. One of the fastest growing segments in gym memberships is people over 65 years of age. Awareness about health and physical activity is probably greater for the Boomers at their age than any other generation before them. As they retire, some Boomers are going into second careers because their physical health is probably much better than generations before them.

They're also thinking about streamlining, simplifying. Sometimes that means downsizing. They were the ones who went for the minivans and the large SUVs like Ford Explorer; but now they have a penchant for the mid-size SUVs like the Escape and the Edge. That appetite for smaller things can be seen in lots of other generations too. So the Boomers are as relevant as they've ever been.

Vaughan

It's one thing to be physically active but to remain a safe driver you have to keep up your cognitive skills too.

Connelly

I think we're a long way off from the average Boomer experiencing any sort of cognitive impairment. With medical advances hopefully it's not inevitable, or it can be postponed even if it is.

You might have heard the quote by Aubrey de Grey, the author who has written about gerontology. He said the first person to live to 150 has probably already been born. On that basis, Boomers are in mid-life with a long way to go.

Instead of thinking you'll drive until you're 82 because you believe you will live to 85 – that becomes a completely different decision if you think you're going to live to 105.

Vaughan

Shouldn't you package up all the safety tech and driver assistance features in new Fords as some kind of Boomer Package and promote it to this aging demographic?

Connelly

Our fundamental effort is to find ways to ensure the freedom, autonomy, and independence that comes from owning and operating your own vehicle. But we don't package these features together as the Boomer package or a package for the aging because people who might have the most use for these don't want to be thought of as old people. We approach it through the concept of universal design. That means we're trying to develop solutions that appeal to all ages so it resonates with you whether you're 71 or 17.

Vaughan

So Boomers don't need the self-driving car yet.

Connelly

We're really trying to focus on technologies that keep the drivers in the seat. We're not looking for a situation where you sit in the passenger seat and you take a nap and wake up at the destination.

But we do know that when it comes to aging, there are some physiological effects that are undeniable. It generally translates into reduced response time, impaired vision, and limited range of motion. We recognize that what it means to be older today is a lot different than it was years ago.

• •

CHAPTER 3

The People Who Can Take Your License Away

Just in case you think the chapter title is too alarmist, here's a list of the people and institutions that can have the means or the motivation to take you off the road forever:

- Your driver-licensing agency
- Your physician
- Your optometrist
- A law enforcement officer
- A Medical Advisory Board
- Your family
- Your friends
- And in many places, an anonymous tipster.

Yes, there are places where an anonymous telephone tip can start the process that leads directly to you losing your license. Police in towns and cities in both Canada and the United States are urging residents to anonymously report elderly motorists they feel are no longer fit to drive.

But when you look at that list, the physician is the one that has the real power.

What is Mandatory Reporting?

In all of Canada and most of the United States, physicians are required by law to report patients they suspect are medically unfit to drive. This legal requirement to report any patient they believe is unfit to drive also applies, in most places, to optometrists and other health care providers.

It's called mandatory reporting and a lot of doctors don't like it one bit. Some believe it's the worst thing that can happen to a doctor-patient relationship. Besides, the typical general practitioner lacks specific training to make this difficult decision because there are no consistent or precise instructions.

And even where such reporting is not mandatory, physicians have been found legally liable when they failed to report a patient who was later determined to have caused harm to others as a result of medical impairment at the wheel.

Few people seem to realize that mandatory reporting means that a routine trip to the doctor's office for a check-up can result in a temporary or permanent driving license suspension.

A Patchwork of Renewal Standards

On top of the confusing and controversial issue of mandatory reporting, the rules and the procedures about renewing an older driver's license are all over the map. In the U.S. and Canada, it's a state or provincial responsibility and the standards vary enormously. The American Automobile Association, which has done great work on this whole issue, summed it up this way: "Safety and Mobility Crisis Looms for Aging Baby Boomers."

Few drivers plan for retirement from driving but surveys have shown that on average, men outlive their driving careers by 6.2 years and women by 9.4 years.

The Triple A says that licensing standards for Seniors are inadequate and inconsistent and finds the states (and let me add the provinces) are not doing enough to prepare for the flood of older drivers that will be behind the wheel in the coming years.

No automobile association would agree with their members having their car keys taken away just because they reach a certain age; that would kill their business. Nor do they argue that older drivers should simply be turned loose on their own say-so.

The Triple A recommends that the states (and again, I'm adding provinces) should screen all drivers applying for new or renewed licenses, to ensure they are medically and functionally fit to drive. They don't want to alienate their older members so they take the position that everybody should be screened "medically and functionally."

How do you do that? You need mandatory eye exams and in-person testing. How much testing? Is it a simple written test or a real, on the road examination? They leave that up in the air but sound the warning: "If remedies aren't put in place today, we can expect a significant rise in highway safety deaths in the years ahead. That should concern all of us, young and old alike."

AAA is committed to making sure that mature drivers are able to continue driving as long as safely possible and sees a much bigger role for physicians in determining who is fit to drive. They want Medical Advisory Boards established in every state (and I'll add province) to conduct individual case reviews and provide input to policy development.

The Triple A recommends creating "standard reporting laws that provide civil immunity for clinicians, law enforcement and licensing personnel who report people they believe may be medically unfit to drive."

"It's unfortunate that healthcare professionals who believe a patient may be medically unfit to drive in a safe manner do not relay this information to their state Department of Motor Vehicles to spur further screening," said Kissinger. "Doctors are well positioned to ensure their patients are fit to drive safely, yet they are fearful of being sued or losing patients if they take actions to protect others on the road. That has to change."

We're going to get into the details of "Functional Driver Assessments" shortly, but in the meantime, check what the license renewal standards are where you live.

It would fill this entire book to list them for each and every jurisdiction in Canada and the United States but fortunately it has been done for you online. So here's your next homework assignment.

There is a searchable database showing each State and Province's Driver Licensing Policies and Practices affecting older and medically-at-risk drivers. It's from a project that was funded by the AAA Foundation for Traffic Safety, Transport Canada, and the Ontario Neurotrama Foundation.

••

HOMEWORK ASSIGNMENT

It's time to go back to the computer and punch in:

http://lpp.seniordrivers.org/lpp/index.cfm?selection=visionreqs

Click on the drop-down list to see how each state or province addresses the topic of interest to you.

This should keep you busy for a while and it will give you a good idea of what you'll be up against at renewal time. But remember these standards are changing and getting tougher all the time.

••

Identifying Medically-at-Risk Drivers

As you discovered it's a patchwork of license requirements for older drivers. Requirements for license renewal depend on where you live. There's also no agreement on reporting practices, appeals processes or options for restricted licenses.

In all of Canada and most of the United States physicians are required to report patients they suspect are medically unfit to drive. Other jurisdictions in the U.S and Europe do not require their physicians to make such judgments.

Everyone seems to agree that the focus should be on identifying medically-at-risk drivers regardless of age. But there's no accepted methodology for assessing a person's capabilities for continued safe driving.

For example should diabetics be subject to mandatory reporting?

Dangers of Diabetes - Hypoglycemic Driving

In 2009 near Hamilton, Ontario a motorist caused a crash killing three people when he went into diabetic shock. An investigation by Ontario's ombudsman André Marin concluded that the dangers caused by uncontrolled or unaware hypoglycemia should be taken as seriously as drunk driving.

"I think it is as serious as impaired driving, there's no doubt about it. People pass out at the wheel, completely pass out, turning their car into an unguided missile," Marin said.

The driver at fault, Allan Maki who has Type 1 diabetes regulated with insulin, was tried and convicted of dangerous driving causing death yet he continued to hold a valid driver's license for 18 months after the fatal crash.

"In the case of Maki, the accident occurred in 2009," Marin said. "He started having episodes of uncontrolled hypoglycemia as early as 2002. So there's a lag of seven years. And then after he's arrested, charged, (the ministry didn't) pull his record, his driver's license for a year and a half. There's something wrong with that system."

Marin said doctors have "failed" in their duty to report drivers with uncontrolled hypoglycemia.

"Our legislation is full of requirements on doctors to report patients in certain circumstances. It's been here since 1968. It should be done in a much more rigorous, methodical fashion and not allowed to languish," Marin said.

"The medical community doesn't seem to be catching on to their obligation to report back to government and the ministry sometimes gets the information and doesn't act on it. I think that vehicles are missiles and in the hands of drivers with unaware hypoglycemia or uncontrolled hypoglycemia, those missiles are turning out to be uncontrolled and a huge danger to the public. There's no one person or one body that should shoulder the entire responsibility, but having doctors do their duty is the first step."

The ombudsman's office pointed to studies which show 25 per cent of people with diabetes have an inability to recognize when their blood sugar is low, a condition referred to as "hypoglycemic unawareness." It also says in 2010 there were 17,456 drivers with diabetes in Ontario, 7,336 of which are insulin dependent.

Marin said his probe revealed a "litany" of inconsistencies, errors and bureaucratic failures in the province's system for reporting and monitoring drivers with potentially dangerous medical conditions.

"Right now, what is happening in Ontario is bureaucratic calamity mired by general chaos. The forms are outdated. Medical information is not current to support those forms. Forms, which (police say), were sent to the ministry don't arrive . . . (and) the medical community doesn't seem to be catching onto their obligations to report back to government. And the ministry sometimes gets the information and doesn't act on it."

Realistic, Objective Testing Standards Ahead?

Requiring doctors to report patients puts enormous pressure on them, especially when they have increasing numbers of older patients with chronic conditions. They have the legal responsibility but nobody has given the physicians valid tools to determine who is and who is not safe to drive. The reason is the tools haven't been developed.

A big, multi-year, multi-million dollar program has been put together by various governments and health institutions in Canada, to develop the screening tools front-line physicians need to assess driving risk in an accurate, fair, and just manner.

It's called Candrive - Canadian Driving Research Initiative for Vehicular Safety for the Elderly. It's mostly paid for by Transport Canada and the Province of Ontario.

They have signed up about 1,000 elderly volunteers in Canada, Australia, and New Zealand. These volunteers have agreed to provide the researchers with all their medical records and even to get their vehicles wired up so the researchers know everything about where, when, and how they're driving.

Realistic, Objective Testing Standards Ahead?

Candrive is setting out to do two main things:

1. Identify drivers with early evidence of increasing risk, who can benefit from retraining or customized licensing, and direct them to such programs.
2. Identify those who have medical and functional impairments that preclude them from safe driving, cancel their licenses, and help them find alternate means of transportation.

In the meantime, doctors have the power to decide when someone should stop driving. We just don't exactly know how they decide.

A physician's main diagnostic tools (medical history and physical examination) are designed to detect disease, not to evaluate safe driving. As a result, people who are medically and functionally unfit to drive remain on the road while other drivers may have their licenses unfairly or prematurely revoked.

Sometimes family members ask a doctor to revoke a relative's driving privileges. A physician may only see an older driver for short periods of time each year, while the driver's family may be in the car when he or she is driving and may notice frightening symptoms.

Families can express their concerns to a physician but cannot order that a license to be taken away. The doctor has to make that call.

Should older drivers be tested on an annual basis? Candrive won't answer that question yet and doesn't plan to until they develop accurate screening tools for physicians to use.

Warning Signs, Red Flags

In the meantime, Candrive states there are some warning signs that indicate that drivers should voluntarily seek their doctor's opinion regarding their driving safety:

- If a driver finds that he or she is getting lost or needing more directions from passengers.
- If a driver is causing other drivers to drive defensively or other drivers are demonstrating frequent signs of irritation with him or her (e.g. horn honking).
- If there have been recent motor vehicle crashes, minor fender-benders in parking lots, increased near-misses, or traffic citations.
- If family or friends become unwilling to be passengers.
- If the driver is losing confidence in his or her own driving ability and becoming on the road.

Testing Standards Depend on Where you Live

Whether you volunteer to talk to your doctor or not, you will likely face a mandatory driving fitness examination of some form, depending on where you live. It could come up automatically when you reach age 80 in some places or it could come up because a doctor or optometrist reported your medical condition to the government. How they report depends on the jurisdiction in which they practise.

And as I mentioned, even where such reporting is not mandatory, physicians may still be found legally liable if they fail to report a patient who is later determined to have caused harm to others as a result of medical impairment at the wheel.

As you learned on your homework assignment when you checked out the licensing requirements on the seniordrivers.org website, in most places both physicians and optometrists are required to report to the Registrar of Motor Vehicles any patient, age 16 or over, who may be suffering from a medical/visual condition that could impair driving ability.

As a rule, if that medical report indicates that you don't meet the medical standards for driving, your driver's license will be suspended. A notice of suspension will be sent to you, along with a letter telling you what medical information is required to have your case reconsidered.

As an alternative, in some states and provinces, you may be required to be assessed at a driving assessment centre. That means a formal driving evaluation with an Occupational Therapist at a government-approved assessment centre.

Functional Driving Assessments

The components of a comprehensive driving evaluation are an in-clinic medical assessment and an on-road driving evaluation. It takes 3-4 hours to complete and must be performed by a qualified Occupational Therapist and a Qualified Driving Instructor.

In-clinic:

Medical history – general medical information, previous and current medical concerns, lifestyle issues.

Physical assessment – relating to range of motion, joint movement, strength, sensation, balance, reaction time, mobility.

Vision assessment – a basic visual screening.

Cognitive and perceptual assessments – tests relating to visual perception, concentration, reaction time, speed of decision-making.

On-road:

An in-car examination, including basic driving manoeuvres.

All this is the subject of the next chapter.

....

FEATURE INTERVIEW

Shawn Marshall, MD MSc FRCPC

Principal co-investigator for the Canadian Driving Research Initiative for Vehicular Safety in the Elderly (Candrive)

Vaughan

How do doctors generally feel about the legal requirement that they report on their patients who they believe might be unfit to drive for medical reasons?

Marshall

There have been studies done at the local and national level on mandatory reporting and physicians have said it negatively affects the physician/patient relationship. Physicians don't like reporting. That's an important reason why

Candrive was funded. We're developing objective, evidence-based tools to assist physicians in making the right decision.

Vaughan

If doctors don't like mandatory reporting, does that lead to under-reporting?

Marshall

I think there's good evidence to suggest that. It's a controversial topic. In the province of Ontario, where there is mandatory reporting, it's absolutely true that there's evidence that physicians are under-reporting.

Vaughan

If I thought my doctor was going to blow the whistle on me, I'd change doctors fast.

Marshall

That's the unfortunate thing. You'd agree that you wouldn't want to be unsafe but at the same time, as a patient, you'd also agree that wow – if I'm not able to drive that's going to have a major negative impact on my life. That's why my co-lead, Dr. Malcolm Man-Son-Hing, and I got into this in the first place, a decade ago. It was around this problem. How do we find objective evidence to identify those who are at increased risk? We need to help physicians and health care providers to identify those older drivers who might be medically at risk for driving, with objective measures that will be accepted by physicians, patients, the general public, and administrators.

Vaughan

Some doctors have said 65 and out. In other words, mandatory retirement from driving for everyone when they hit that age. Do you agree?

Marshall

No. Obviously everyone wants to continue driving and if they can, they should. First of all, it's not about age; it's about the medical condition and the health effects. By identifying things in an objective manner, we can look at what can keep drivers on the road longer. We can look at what interventions might be effective to keep them on the road longer. Driver refreshment can be effective. There's evidence that conditional licensing programs can be effective. Especially in rural areas that's very important.

Vaughan

Why has this study taken so long? You're five years into it and you haven't delivered the goods yet.

Marshall

We think we're pretty close. But it is an international study involving 7 sites and over 1000 older drivers. We study outcomes and the most important one is at-fault collisions.

The minimum age for entry to our study group is 70 and the average age is about 77. Now, after 4 or 5 years we now have the average age above 80 in our study.

We have had to wait for the results to come in. We need those outcomes, the at-fault collisions, to do the assessments. Sometimes collisions are just a matter of being at the wrong place at the wrong time but it's the at-fault collisions that everyone would agree must be avoided. Now we're looking at numbers we project will be enough for at-fault collisions that were due to health reasons. Now we will be able to determine what are these risk factors.

Vaughan

The Canadian Medical Association, of which you're a member, has published a 150-page Drivers Guide for Physicians, on the evaluation of fitness to drive. If they've done it already, aren't you just reinventing the wheel?

Marshall

No, because the evidence on which decisions are made by physicians through the CMA guide is thin. If you read the guidelines for physicians, they say things such as 'you should evaluate or monitor' this person but it doesn't give you a line in the sand that allows you to make an individual decision. We're looking for objective evidence that this person is at increased risk so that when you see this or define this, it means this person is at increased risk and this is how we can help them.

CHAPTER 4

Pass the Test

Okay, you have now arrived at the point where you will have to prove that you still have the goods to be a safe driver. You're about to be the subject of a Functional Driving Assessment.

There are a number of possible reasons why you are here including:

Your doctor recommended it.

As you know, almost everywhere your physician (and optometrist, psychologist and psychiatrist, if you have one) has a legal responsibility to notify the motor vehicle office if he or she believes you have a condition that makes you unsafe to drive. You also know that many physicians under-report, knowing the drastic consequences of putting an "unsafe-to-drive" opinion in the hands of the licensing people.

Many physicians explain to the patient the medical reasons why they *might* be unsafe to drive and tell him or her that instead of "sending the letter," they'd like the patient to get a prompt, second opinion from a Certified Driver Assessment Center.

It's a veiled threat but you should gratefully accept it. Your physician is sticking his or her neck out for you, so follow the advice and book the Functional Driving Assessment appointment at once.

Your doctor ordered it.

Legally qualified medical practitioners are aware of their "mandatory reporting" responsibilities. They know that if their patient has medical and/or psychological conditions that interfere with safe driving, they are obliged to "send the letter." That results in the patient's driver's license being suspended or considered for suspension. Unless you decide at that point you wish to "retire" from driving, then the Functional Driving Assessment is your only other option.

Your lawyer told you to.

This probably means you've waited too long and have been involved in a collision as a driver and you have been charged with a violation and maybe sued. Your lawyer might be trying to spread the blame to someone else. (See mandatory reporting above.)

A concerned friend, business associate, or family member talked you into it.

This might be the best reason of all. People who know you best may have observed things about your driving that make them nervous. Don't get all angry and resentful – get proactive. Book yourself a Functional Driving Assessment and find out the facts. If you're a "borderline" case, there is lots of training available to keep you sharp and legal.

The Functional Driving Assessment

You're going to book an appointment with a Driver Assessment and Training Specialist. These are for-profit companies or non-profit organizations made up of people who have academic and clinical qualifications and are certified by the jurisdiction in which you are living.

Their main business is usually providing driver training for people with physical disabilities or serious injuries, who want to drive.

You're there to get an Assessment Report for license eligibility.

Your Clinical Assessment will be done by an occupational therapist (OT), who has specialized expertise in driving assessment and rehabilitation. Your on-the-road assessment will be done by a certified driving instructor with the OT riding along and observing.

Clinical Assessment First

It is about an hour and a half long. You'll get tested for few fairly simple, physical motions and functions, a vision check, and a battery of cognition tests. In other words, they're trying to measure your cognitive and motor skills before they put you behind the wheel.

Once that's over, you'll get an On-Road Evaluation, which is conducted by the driving instructor with the occupational therapist observing from the back seat.

If your license has already been suspended due to "mandatory reporting" you, of course, are not allowed to drive to the assessment and must be driven there by a family member or friend. You will have to apply for and receive a one- day temporary license for this assessment and bring it with you. You'll have to bring in a list of any medication you're on and the glasses you use for reading and/or driving. You may also have medical reports and paperwork from the motor vehicles department.

What Results Can You Expect?

Before we get into the details of the testing, let's be realistic about your chances of passing it. If your doctor has triggered the suspension of your driving license by "mandatory reporting," you can be pretty sure he or she has had good reasons for doing so. In that case, experience shows that while you're certainly entitled to challenge the doctor's judgment by taking the test and passing it – I don't like your chances.

I volunteered for a number of full Functional Driving Assessments to see what they're like. Fortunately, I passed them all and what I can tell you from my experience, is that the Occupational Therapist and the driving instructor are on your side. They have high professional and ethical standards and will not pass you under any circumstances, if they determine that you're a menace on the roads.

However, they are both in the "rehabilitation" business and if they determine responsibly that you are close enough to the legal standards that training and practise will get you there – that's what they'll recommend. You won't get your license back that day but they may be able to point you in that direction.

But back to why I don't like your chances if your doctor's "mandatory reporting" has resulted in your license suspension. I haven't seen any official statistics on this – if there are any – but through conversations with OTs it's become clear to me that in very few cases is it proven the doctor got it wrong.

I'm almost positive your doctor told you why it was necessary for you to retire from driving when he or she told you about the "mandatory report." There are exceptions, doctors aren't perfect but I'd say the odds are strongly against you.

Now let's say you're taking the Functional Driving Assessment not because your license has been pulled but because your doctor strongly recommended it. In this case – again no official statistics – but it looks like there is less than a 50/50 chance you'll get a pass on the evaluation. Some doctors don't want to be the bearer of bad news to a longtime patient and some genuinely aren't sure and want a second opinion. You have a chance – prepare yourself for Assessment Day and give it your best shot. More about that later.

The Occupational Therapist (O.T.)

Don't be afraid of taking a Functional Driver Assessment. Let's say you were smart enough to realize it yourself, or you were diplomatically told by a friend or family member that your driving isn't what it used to be. In that case, I strongly recommend you book yourself in for a driving evaluation with the intention of rehabilitation work, if needed.

From everything I've seen, I'm very confident you'll get the straight goods from the OT and the driving instructor on how you shape up as a safe driver. The evaluation will probably cost you five or six hundred bucks but it is money well spent. We talked about it earlier but if you've had a few close calls on the road or in the parking lot and especially if you've noticed people aren't comfortable as your passengers, then do the right thing and sign yourself up for evaluation.

It's hard to say what the pass rate of this approach will be because there are so few people who have had the sense to "volunteer" for evaluation. But I've done it and will continue to do it every few years in the future.

What Happens If Your License Has Already Been Suspended?

When you walk in, you're likely to be handed a Client Agreement form, which begins with your name, address, birth date and driver's license type and number. Then you have to give Informed Consent.

In the Consent section, you have to sign off on the fact that you understand the purpose of the assessment is to determine your potential as a driver in view of illness, disability, medical condition, whatever. You agree to both the Clinical Assessment and the On the Road Assessment and agree that the result of either could be "driving cessation."

Next, there's usually some kind of Assumption of Risk, where you release the testing company from any liabilities if you crash the car in your driving test.

Next up; the Disclosure section where you agree that the results of this assessment – whatever they may be – will be sent to your physician and to the motor vehicles department. At this point you'll probably wish that you'd volunteered for assessment and some retraining a couple of years ago. Then the official evaluation begins.

The Clinical Evaluation

Now you sit down in a quiet office with an occupational therapist. If you have a family member with you, then the OT will probably want that person to be alongside you.

The discussion usually begins with medical history-taking, focussing on the physician's report – stroke, heart disease, diabetes? Then you'll be asked for a summary of the frequency of medications taken.

Then, into a discussion of driving patterns and concerns. How often do you drive, when, where? Any concerns? Are you comfortable, confident? Drive at night? Drive on highways? Any crashes? Close calls? They're very interested in any driving anxiety issues you might have. The OT will be looking for reactions from the family member too.

Next up will be mild testing of physical abilities. Raise your arms, lower your arms, turn your head, lift your leg, point your toes – that sort of thing. Then a couple of strength tests – grip this, squeeze that. Then a vision test and a peripheral vision test.

Now we come to the cognitive stuff. This is what really counts; it's basically to test the thinking skills you need for driving. The OT wants to know about your cognitive functioning, perception, vision, driver insight and judgment.

Cognitive Assessment

Now if you remember, back in Chapter 3 we talked about the big multi-year, multi-million dollar Candrive study that is trying to develop evidence-based tools that healthcare people can use to fairly test driving ability – particularly on the mental side of things.

They haven't come up with that "line in the sand" yet and in the meantime, various assessment centers use various combinations of tests to come up with the answer. Probably the best known is the DriveABLE Cognitive Assessment Tool.

DriveABLE is a spin-off company from the University of Alberta which developed both an In-Clinic test and an On-Road test, which assess a driver based on the level of cognitive impairment caused by his or her medical condition.

Some physicians love it and some don't. DriveABLE is a private, for-profit company and doesn't release all its data and scientific conclusions – in other words it doesn't want the competition to get the "secret sauce."

I'm no psychologist but it seemed to be a good test to me so I'll explain a little about how it works. If you don't get DriveABLE you'll get something like it although it might be done with paper and pencil and not be computer-based.

In the DriveABLE test they sit you down in front of a computer and you're asked to complete six tasks, each of which is clearly explained and demonstrated. You get to practice them a couple of times before you have to do them. If you can play the Helicopter Game, even at a slow speed on your computer, you'll have no problem at all with the tests.

The premise is that driving requires the complex interaction of several mental abilities. The DCAT - the DriveABLE Cognitive Assessment Tool - is composed of six tasks that predict whether you would fail an on-road test because of a decline in your cognitive abilities such as memory, attention, judgment, decision-making, and identification of hazardous situations.

The result returned by the DCAT is a score between 1% and 99% and reflects the Predicted Probability of Failing an On-Road Evaluation, 1 being least likely and 99 being the most likely to fail the on-road.

I am happy to report that my score was 1% but that's not why I like the test. It seemed very comprehensive and maybe a little less subjective than evaluator opinion. Also it produces a number for each of the following: Motor Speed/Control, Span of Attention Field, Spatial Judgment and Decision Making, Executive Function, and Identification of Driving Situations.

You can Google all those terms if you're puzzled but the DCAT shows if you have vision, memory, and the ability to keep track of more than one thing at once. And as I said, it produces a score – a number. Doctors love numbers as a diagnostic result because it seems to keep the guesswork out.

DriveABLE is a for-profit company and the DCAT software is licensed for use to healthcare organizations and licensing authorities. They don't give out free samples so you can't practise at home. But, in a way, it's similar to a vision or hearing test; you cannot study to pass it. DriveABLE does not measure your driving skills; it assesses cognitive functions.

If you want to practise tests like this, just Google "brain test" and you'll find dozens you can play for free. One of the very best sites to visit is www.aarp.org. AARP is a non-profit, non-partisan organization that helps people 50 and older improve the quality of their lives. Click on the Games button and find Brain Games. If you can handle any of these you'll have no trouble with DCAT.

On Road Evaluation

You can flame out on the cognitive test so badly that you won't be given the On Road test because it's clear the brain's not working well enough and you'd be a hazard on the road. But that doesn't happen very often and let's assume it's not going to happen to you. So the driving test is next.

You're put behind the wheel of a dual-brake car – that means the instructor can hit the brakes on his or her side of the car if you're really screwing up. In the test, you are given simple, explicit driving directions well in advance. They don't worry about minor errors that might come up because you're not familiar with the vehicle and only "competence-defining errors defined by the research are scored."

They're looking for the big mistakes – not looking, wandering across lanes, severe anxiety, confused thinking – that kind of thing. You're compared with normal healthy drivers in your same age range.

I'd recommend that anyone taking this test should brush up in advance, if possible, with another Certified Driving Instructor. They are going to be able to point out the little things that might accumulate to produce a bad score. Things like making complete stops – not rolling stops – exactly at the white line and not in front of or behind. And they're sticklers for making shoulder turns on every lane change – checking the mirror is not enough.

Anyway, I came through this one okay too. The good news; my "driving performance revealed no evidence that driving competence is outside the range of normal, healthy drivers."

Well, that wouldn't exactly get me a seat in Formula One but the conclusion was; "Driving cessation is NOT indicated." That's what I was looking for.

Any Second Chances?

Don't forget that the results from your unsuccessful test are going to your doctor and to the motor vehicles department and neither wants to see you put up a string of "Driving Cessation Indicated" scores.

But as I mentioned, the people who conducted your test are in the training and rehabilitation business. I believe they will level with you. If you are a borderline case in the On Road portion, they might prescribe a rehabilitative training program to try to get you back to safe driving. It would include on-the-road training and assistance to get you ready for the road test portion of another Functional Driving Assessment.

However, if you blew the cognitive test badly then it is definitely time to turn in the keys.

The Rules Are Changing

Certain provinces and states are working on changing the license-renewal process of those aged 80 and above.

In Ontario, for example, those drivers will have to pass a test every two years. This procedure used to take about three hours and would include a written test. In its place will be a vision test, a review of the subject's driving record, a refresher course in a classroom setting, plus an in-class screening component, administered in the form of two short exercises.

Here's a sample test.

Ontario's Age 80 and Above License Renewal Program:
Group Education Session (GES) In-Class
Screening Component: Practice Samples

Part A
Instructions

1. On a separate sheet of paper, draw a large circle.
2. Put all the numbers in to make it look like the face of a clock.
3. Draw the hands of the clock to show ten minutes after eleven.
4. Stop when completed.

Part B
Instructions:

1. Look at the letters below.
2. Whenever you see an "H", cross it out
3. Stop when completed.

B D A H C F B H D E H D A F H I C H F H
D H C E H I H G D H G E B H E G H I H C
C G D H C B A H G D E H C H B E H D G H
H C D H F H C D H B H D H F A C H C H F
E B H G F B H F A H E B G H G F E H D B
G E H G H D E H C G H D H E B A H F B H

Then, based on the results, a road test may be required. An aging advocacy group in Canada responded to the changes by stating, "Two-thirds of Senior drivers have good or very good visual, auditory, and cognitive capabilities, according to Stats Canada. It's the small portion of elderly drivers that struggles with these things, which gives the whole group a bad name. It's a difficult topic that affects one of the fastest-growing population segments. The most common response is 'take away their license,' but that's not the solution to this complex problem."

Practice, Practice, Practice

The licensing authorities always say their aim is to keep Seniors driving for as long as they can safely do so. No matter where you live, a Functional Driving Assessment or a Supplemental Driving Performance Evaluation (SDPE) is in your future at some point. I've explained what it's all about but there is a 30-page study guide prepared by the California Department of Motor Vehicles that sets out the test and the ways to prepare it in detail.

The study guide is available for free online and I strongly suggest you try it out. It is found at www.dmv.ca.gov/pubs/dl956.pdf

Local Drive Tests Could be Part of the Solution

A few jurisdictions have a program designed to license drivers only for local roads and under specific conditions.

This licensing program examines drivers on familiar streets near their homes. Drivers who pass this Local Drive Test (LDT) are then issued a restricted license that permits them to drive only in the general area where they were tested. Additional restrictions, such as time of day and road conditions, could also apply.

The State of Iowa ran an experimental LDT program between 2005 and 2008. They signed up 205 Seniors, with an average age of 85. In the three years, that group had a lower overall crash rate than all the rest of licensed drivers in the state. In other words, LDT-licensed drivers were as safe, or safer, than the general population, while still enjoying a good level of mobility.

FEATURE INTERVIEW

With John Sheard, President of DriveLab

John Sheard has more than 25 years experience as a hands-on rehabilitation, business specialist. He has managed over 60,000 cases involving personal injury caused by violent crimes, motor vehicle crashes, industrial accidents and disease process. John's expert opinions in Vocational Rehabilitation are accepted by the Ontario WSIAT (Workplace Safety & Insurance Appeals Tribunal).

DriveLab provides graded exposure to driving, for people who have physical, cognitive, emotional, or developmental disabilities, as well as to Seniors who require assistance in maintaining their driver status.

Vaughan

As you know, I went through a Functional Driver Assessment with DriveLab. The registered occupational therapist who put me through the clinical assessment was Elana Korman, who has a Masters of Science degree. The testing was thorough and fair and Elana certainly has the medical training and the people skills to do an evidence-based assessment. Fortunately, I passed but she told me, although I took the test voluntarily, had she determined that I had a condition that made me unfit to drive a car, she would have informed the licensing authorities at once.

Sheard

I wasn't joking with you when you told me you wanted to do the test. If you hadn't passed, we would have notified the licensing office. This is a serious business. You are talking about the risk a health care professional is taking to tell someone in authority that you are safe to drive a 4,000 pound piece of metal down a high-speed highway and not kill anybody. That's not taken lightly, believe me.

Vaughan

It is a major responsibility that's placed on your shoulders.

Sheard

When I first started this business, I had a hard time getting any insurance anywhere. They looked at it and called it a non-standard product. They didn't know how to write it. They'd never seen it before. They didn't know how to write the risk. What we did 25 years ago was a service that nobody had really heard of. Today it is becoming more important and as a consequence, more visible. Today it's important to do this kind of work – period.

Vaughan

Physicians nearly everywhere have a legal obligation to report patients whom they deem to be unfit, to the licensing office. That's the mandatory reporting. Do you believe physicians follow that rule 100% of the time?

Sheard

I'd be surprised. It would be unlikely. People begin to decline cognitively at 55 years old. On that basis, everyone over 55 years old might theoretically be considered an at-risk driver. By that measure, everyone should be reported at 55 years old, which doesn't happen obviously.

I think it's a prickly decision for a doctor. I don't think many doctors want to get embroiled in that kind of situation. We live in a car culture. Mobility is very important. Take their license away and many couldn't get to the store. It's almost like you're being sentenced to live your life at home.

Vaughan

That's why Functional Driver Assessment is relied on.

Sheard

The occupational therapist doing that kind of work is at the centre point. The Occupational Therapist seems to be taking the visible responsibility for that decision. In point of fact, it is the government, as advised by a Medical Advisory Committee, which has the ultimate decision.

Vaughan

Do you think there should mandatory testing?

Sheard

I don't think the elderly driver should be treated any differently. What about a seventeen-year-old kid who has had a head injury from a car crash? Why is he any different from an elderly driver? Or a trucker who is fifty years old and has had a stroke? Why is the elderly driver penalized and treated any differently? I don't think they should be treated differently. I think anyone who has a medical or psychological condition that would imperil their ability to drive should be subject to some form of scrutiny and this is what we do.

Vaughan

Are you going easy on elderly people?

Sheard

I see some horrible drivers on the road – drivers my age. Some elderly drivers have a problem at a stoplight. They can't turn left. They can't process the information. That's what it is – visual information processing. One of these days, I'll face the same thing. I know I won't be able to drive forever. I'll face that. It's the aging process. I think people are very worried about facing this kind of a situation because after all, it kind of signals the beginning of the end.

Vaughan

Can that day be delayed?

Sheard

The reality is that it's not just the elderly who are at risk, but the entire Boomer generation. They just don't appreciate it yet. They will pay a small fortune to get their hair done. They will pay a small fortune for pets. They will pay money to go to Bingo or the casino. None of those are life essentials but transportation is. Really, people should be prepared to pay driver rehabilitation specialists for the services needed to preserve their opportunity to drive. Maybe programmes like ours would help extend their safe driving life.

Vaughan

Is there funding available for your assessments?

Sheard

I know that you have focused on the elderly but you would be surprised what other populations need help. When we work with people who are fearful of driving after a crash, insurance companies sometimes cover our work. They should cover it all the time because our work is a risk-minimization strategy for them. Our job is to help people avoid a second crash and you would be surprised how often a second or third crash happens. If I talked to a Claims Manager, he or she would see us as a cost to be avoided. If I spoke to the Vice President of Underwriting, he or she would see us as a tool to avoid another crash or loss.

CHAPTER 5

Who's in Charge Here? The Data or the Driver?

Automated driving becomes ever closer. Continental, the German automotive-systems supplier, has received a license from the State of Nevada to begin testing automated vehicles on Nevada roads. The test vehicles havespecial red license plates and must have a driver at the wheel, just in case things go wrong.

In getting the license, Continental revealed a plan that puts Fully Automated driving on high-speed highways in 2025. Partially Automated driving comes first in 2016 and Highly Automated driving could happen by 2020.

Here's what the terms mean: Fully Automated means the driver does nothing and the cars race along highways at 130km/h. Highly Automated is basically the same but at lower speeds. Partially Automated is here now and it means the car drives itself in stop-and-go traffic jams at speeds below 30 km/h. With both the "Partial" and "High" levels of automation, however, the driver must be able to take control of the vehicle at all times.

The example the engineers trot out is of course the use of autopilots in aviation. Pilots would never say they "set it and forget it" but automated systems control aircraft en route and maintain proper separation from other aircraft with little or no pilot input. Automotive engineers say the same technology can take the monotony out of long-distance journeys on major highways.

The Nevada test vehicles will, for the most part, use systems and sensors that Continental already supplies to manufacturers. There are four short-range radar sensors (two at the front, two at the rear), one long-range radar sensor, and a stereo camera. The vehicle is able to track all objects as they enter into the sensors' field of view. The information is then processed and passed on to a "Motion Domain Controller," which sends signals to the engine, the brakes, and the steering.

So if things work out as planned, by 2020 you should be able to eat breakfast, read the newspaper or surf the web as you drive along. The 2016 automated stop-and-go driving is ahead of schedule – it's just a matter of rolling it out in more new cars. The promise of all this is that automatically controlled vehicles will be safer because of the interaction between the vehicle and its environment. Autonomous cars will react faster and more reliably than humans are capable of doing.

Eventually, automated vehicles will also be able communicate with each other. They will be able to alert other autonomous cars that there's a car being driven in a dangerous way ahead of them, and react. An automated car would know that there was someone approaching unseen from a side street at a high rate of speed and do an emergency stop.

The Head of the US National Highway Traffic Safety Administration, David Strickland, said that self-driving cars have the potential to save "thousands and thousands of lives." Strickland says human error played a part in around 90% of the more than 33,000 traffic deaths on American roads in 2010. He called automated vehicles the "next evolutionary step" for cars.

But the technology is only one part of the story of self-driving cars; the other part is the legality of them. What happens when an automated car gets into an accident? – It will happen. Who will be liable for damages? The computer maker, the software, or the driver who wasn't driving? Answering all the legal questions could well delay the automated-driving timetable that hopeful engineers and safety officials are eagerly laying out.

It's Only Code

A little while ago, I had a conversation with Dieter Zetsche, the Daimler CEO. He had arrived at a social event, in connection with the Frankfurt Auto Show, in the back seat of a driverless car. It was the new S-Class Mercedes, in a demonstration of autonomous driving.

I said to him, "You can load all this self-driving technology into an S-Class because they sell for a hundred thousand plus but will this stuff ever reach the lower-priced cars?" He looked at me as though I had a screw loose and said, "Yes, easily. It's only code." Pause. "You know, software."

Writing code is a lot cheaper than bending metal. Zetsche is a man accustomed to spending huge amounts of money. The price tag to develop a new vehicle starts around $1 billion and can run to 5 or 6 bill, if it's an all-new platform with new power trains. You can have rooms and rooms full of software developers in their propeller beanies and not notice the cost in a game like this.

Big Data is a big deal for next-generation cars.

In a new car, there are already hundreds of sensors, connected to microcontrollers that run the engine, brakes, airbags, traction control – the works. It's all "drive by wire" these days. Pressing the accelerator no longer pulls a throttle cable; the steering wheel is no longer directly connected to the wheels. Sensors and data processing are making most of the decisions already and adding a little more "code" will deliver many, many more functions at little extra cost.

Gyroscopes and accelerometers are already in place for anti-rollover systems. GPS is practically standard these days. Ultrasonic systems and radar and stereo cameras are already watching traffic, following lane markers, reading signs, and detecting accidents before they happen. The next thing coming is vehicles that communicate with the driving infrastructure (V2I) and vehicles that communicate with other vehicles (V2V).

The assumption is if you can predict the accident – you can prevent the accident. Well, you can't, but the technology can and it will make the car drive itself out of the way.

Getting vehicles to talk among themselves and communicate with the "cloud" means that whoever is in the vehicle is telling the world a great deal about themselves personally. Like, why were you at this sketchy location at 2:00a.m. And why were you driving so badly? And why do you always buy your jug of milk (or quart of Scotch) at that store when it's cheaper on the next block with the coupon that was just sent to your car?

A great example of how data can be used against you was the way Tesla hung a car reviewer for the *New York Times* out to dry. The reviewer had claimed in print that the all-electric Tesla had run out of juice early and had to be towed home.

However, Tesla lashed back by releasing the raw data from the vehicle, which showed that charging stations had been driven past, that the car was unplugged before it reached full charge, that it had been driven at greater speeds than claimed, and even that the heater had been on high. In other words, the data shot the reviewer's story and his credibility full of holes.

To make the most out of Big Data, vehicles will have to communicate a lot of information about you, whether you like it or not. If you have a plug-in vehicle, the electrical utility will use artificial intelligence programs to manage where and when you plug in, so everyone doesn't plug in at once and crash the aging grid. And when they know your driving habits, they'll know you don't need 30 amps and will only dish out 10 if there's high demand.

Big Data can only deliver big benefits with data-sharing cars. Will it also be a big infringement on our privacy? It sure looks like it. But maybe it's worth it if we get better fuel economy, get stuck less in traffic, and actually have way fewer accidents. It's possible and it costs very little. "It's only code."

Ford's Talking Car

"Hey you, listen up. This is your car talking and I want you to find a safe place and pull over right now. I've just watched your glucose level fall off the scale and I want you to stop and have that snack and juice box before you pass out. And when you pull over, push the recirculation button on the A.C. and don't open the windows. The Oak and Birch pollen levels where you're driving are sky high and that might set off your asthma."

I'm sure they'll pretty-up the script before this goes commercial but Ford is working on making its in-car telematics system, the SYNC – able to monitor health conditions in drivers. They've got a deal with medical-device maker Medtronic to let a driver wearing a Bluetooth-enabled, glucose monitoring device get audible instructions from the car's infotainment system while watching blood glucose levels trend up and down on the dash-mount video screen.

"Hey you, I notice you're still driving. If you don't stop the car now, I'm going turn it off for you. You're two minutes from hypoglycemia."

A stern warning is certainly better than getting lightheaded with blurry vision and maybe passing out. And if SYNC accesses pollen data from a website and automatically changes air-conditioning settings to re-circulate filtered air, asthma and allergy sufferers might avoid coughing and wheezing attacks.

Ford engineers are always talking about their cars as technology platforms while pointing out that young people especially never want to be without their infotainment technology. Right now, you can get a car with SYNC that will recognize about 10,000 voice commands. You can tell the Navi to find you the closest gas station or the one with the cheapest gas and it will direct you there in spoken commands. You can tell the climate control you want the temperature at 21.5 degrees and the satellite radio set on Redneck Channel and you'll get both without an argument. Moving into the health and wellness area with this stuff could be the next big thing for automotive telematics.

It's happening now on smartphones. There are something like 17,000 smartphone, medical and health care apps available and most of them are aimed at consumers, not health-care professionals. Ford thinks people will want to be able to get this information hands-free while they're sitting behind the wheel.

Ford has a few other things going on in health and wellness technologies too. They did a study with the Massachusetts Institute of Technology (MIT) on the relationship between stress and driving performance, which apparently proved that drivers are less stressed if they can get around traffic jams by being directed by SYNC. That's no surprise and now they're looking at other ideas to keep drivers relaxed and under control. Ford hasn't announced a timetable to get the health monitoring into Sync but it can't be far off.

"Okay, Knucklehead, listen up. I see you stopped the car and now your glucose level is getting back to normal. Good. But now I see that your temperature and blood pressure are on the rise. Are you cursing out some other driver? Are you getting a little too aggressive out there? Settle down or I'm turning off the engine again."

Now they just have to work on the scripts.

Beat the Traffic Lights

Audi is working on advanced traffic-light recognition technology, to get you through the city on more green lights.

Audi Online traffic-light information uses in-car Internet to establish a link between the car and the traffic light network, via the central traffic computer in a town or city.

It takes in the automated traffic-light change sequences in the vicinity and then tells you the speed to drive, in order to pass through the light while it's green. If you're already stuck at a red light, the system counts down the time remaining until green and connects to the car's

Start-Stop function, to ensure the engine is switched on five seconds before green.

Audi says the system is ready to go but it needs government approval and cooperation.

Big Daddy? No, Big Data. The Internet of Things

IBM and the US telecommunications giant, AT&T are combining on an Internet of Things partnership. Cisco has tied up with Swiss security firm AGT International in a similar venture and Google and Microsoft and even Amazon are also taking a shot at what's thought to be a $600-billion pie.

The idea is to sell services to government agencies, to integrate and analyze huge volumes of data that are produced by cars, cell phones, road sensors, utility meters, transit gates, security cameras – you name it. Analyzing the movement of people should improve traffic management, parking allocation, and the speedy arrival of emergency services.

Rick Qualman, a vice president at IBM said, "The new collaboration with AT&T will offer insights from crowdsourcing, mobile applications, sensors and analytics on the cloud, enabling all organizations to better listen, respond, and predict."

Cisco and AGT have similar plans. They want to build a traffic-management system that incorporates sensors embedded in pavements, license plate-reading systems, social media feeds, and video cameras to, "identify, respond to, and resolve," traffic incidents in real time.

Some people are worried about a "traffic management" system that reads license plate numbers and integrates social media. It's the Snowden Problem. Since Edward Snowden exposed the NSA's habit of eavesdropping on governments and Google and other big web companies, many people fear the Internet of Things will further compromise their privacy and their security.

No, no, says IBM; "Smarter cities, cars, homes, machines, and consumer devices will drive the growth of the Internet of Things, unleashing a wave of new possibilities for data gathering, predictive analytics, and automation."

In other words, it's part of a large trend in which city, state, and federal agencies use sensors to monitor the smallest aspects of everyday urban life.

The Cisco / AGT partners want to use sensors embedded in roads, which is along the same lines as one of Google's plans for self-driving cars. Google's eventual hope is that sensors placed at regular intervals on highways can help guide driverless cars to their destinations.

This is the smart-roads approach. A recent example of this is a Volvo research project that placed magnets eight inches below a roadway, to help cars determine their position.

However, magnetic sensors don't come cheap. Some estimates say $40,000 a mile, minimum, plus maintenance. Add that to 4-million miles of roads and costs mount up. Plus, all the gear needed in Google's self-driving car is around $250,000.

Driver-assistance technologies are here now. Self-driving technology and the physical and legal infrastructure to support it are still a long, long way off. I think we'll all need valid driving licenses well into the future.

A Relatively Easy Step Toward a Crash-free Future

The car that drives itself is still a science experiment but there are components of "autonomous driving" that several carmakers sell today. Auto-braking is one of them and it is a big step forward for road safety. In fact, new crash-test regulations mean that Autonomous Emergency Braking (AEB) technology will soon be in most, if not all, cars.

Accident research shows that about 90% of all crashes happen at speeds below 20mph (32kmh). These are the rear end collisions in slow traffic or at a stoplight when a driver isn't paying enough attention. Maybe the car in front stops suddenly and when you notice, you slam on the brakes but it's too late. There's damage to both cars but it's also the slow-speed crashes that bring about whiplash claims.

A study by the European Commission suggests that widespread adoption of AEB could reduce accidents by more than 25%. Volvo was first to introduce AEB on its XC60, in 2008, and now nearly every manufacturer has a version.

Of course they all have different names and different characteristics. For Audi, it's "Pre-Sense Front Plus," while Honda uses, "Collision Mitigation Brake System." For Mercedes, it's "Collision Prevention Assist" and for Volvo, "City Safety."

Certain versions also work from higher speeds and can even detect pedestrians and apply the brakes if an impact is imminent. But only a tiny fraction of the cars on the road have any kind of AEB, even though it is a sure way to minimize collisions, reduce insurance costs and save lives.

· ·

FEATURE INTERVIEW

With Thomas Broberg, Senior Technical Advisor – Safety, Volvo Cars, Gothenburg, Sweden

Vaughan

Is your job to build cars that are safe for Seniors?

Broberg

Volvo is thinking about every driver and of course the driver population will change as we go forward. Baby Boomers are going to live longer and healthier than any generation before, which means there will be a higher percentage of older drivers on the road. I am focussing on elderly drivers;

that's actually my study topic – safety for an aging population. My focus is on how we can further enhance active, safety technology for this category of drivers. If we do something that is good for elderly drivers, we are doing something good for every driver.

Vaughan

But there are a number of active safety systems available in cars today though most people don't seem to know about them.

Broberg

This is one of my hot topics that I am currently writing on. There may actually be quite a few technologies already available that would help the elderly drivers and all drivers.

Some elderly people get a new car every couple of years, while some still drive a 15-year-old car. Of course the technical capability of the brand new car and the 10 or 15-year-old car is quite different.

One example is driving when it's dark. A lot of elderly put restrictions on themselves by not driving while it's dark but if you're living in the northern hemisphere, it can get dark at 3 o'clock in the afternoon. There are advanced light systems that steer with the car and some that enable you to have the high beams on all the time and light up the side of the road without blinding the cars coming toward you.

What I have found is that the awareness of some of these driver-support technologies is quite low – not only among the elderly but in general. Blind spot information systems and advanced headlights have been available in cars for quite some time. Autonomous Emergency Braking is available today, including systems that can see pedestrians and bicyclists. The solution is to build cars with senses.

Vaughan

It sounds like you are already.

Broberg

We're getting to the point where we can offer more automated driving in different situations. In a modern car today, you can drive semi-autonomously. With Adaptive Cruise Control, you don't have to regulate your speed. You can follow another vehicle while your car regulates the accelerator and the brake for you. There are some situations where the car can actually steer for you.

We have cars today that can recognize a potential collision, feel if the driver is responding or not, and automatically apply the brakes if necessary.

Vaughan

But people don't ask for these systems or maybe they don't want to pay for them.

Broberg

In our focus groups, we discussed autonomous driving and the acceptance level was quite high. We found there's quite a high acceptance of technology for having the car do things for you. But one concern that came up was that it's advanced electronics, so some feel it would be very difficult and expensive to repair. But it's not.

Vaughan

There are millions of Boomers in retirement age now, with millions more arriving every year. A lot of them have money and would want to buy every active safety technology they can get their hands on. I think some manufacturer should put everything they've got into one model and call it the safest car for Seniors.

Broberg

I'm an engineer and that's a marketing question. But yes, definitely, I think it's a matter of getting the information out there. Show the facts.

· ·

CHAPTER 6

New Technology for Accident Free Driving

Well, accidents do happen and will continue to happen. Accident-free driving is a worthy goal but it's a long way off. However, accident-reduced driving is here right now, as a result of the introduction of new automotive technology.

We've taken a look at new, driver-assistance technology that is still in the future but now let's check out the stuff that's on the market today.

If you've driven the same car for several years and haven't had seat time in the latest models, you don't know what you're missing. Some of the new technology is standard on all cars and SUVs these days but a lot of it is available only as an extra-cost option or is found only in the most expensive vehicles.

This chapter will try to summarize what's available in an understandable way, to help you decide what's worth paying for in your next vehicle purchase. Too many people take the view that because they've driven so many years without it they don't need it now.

What this won't be is a description of what's on every vehicle available. With all the makes and models and trim levels and options, you have well over a thousand choices out there. This chapter is to get you thinking conceptually about the purposes and advantages of safety technology that's currently available and to give you a good sense of where it's going in the near future.

In the course of doing this, we will look more closely at four manufacturers and introduce you to senior engineers at each of them, so you can see the picture through their eyes and find out how it connects to their companies' technology. I'm not saying these companies are necessarily the best in safety technology because all the carmakers are working very hard on this issue and have developed proprietary technology in-house, or have purchased it from a supplier. But within the limitations of a small book, I've chosen four who have been particularly open and helpful.

In the next chapter, we'll go through specific makes and models to check out the advanced safety systems that are available. But let's look at the big picture, to get more familiar with what these systems do, and meet some of the top people who are introducing them to the market.

Analyzing the Need for Safety Assistance

One of the companies at which we will look more closely is Nissan. They call their package of safety technologies the Safety Shield and they conceptualize the need for it in six stages. I think it's a good way to think about the application of technology for accident prevention and mitigation. Here are their six stages.

1. Risk has not yet appeared.

At this stage, they're trying to help the driver to maintain safe driving with assists like Adaptive Cruise Control and 360-degree camera monitors.

2. Risk has appeared.

Now they're trying to help the driver to recover from dangerous conditions to safe driving, with assists like Lane Departure Warning and Lane Departure Prevention.

3. Crash may occur.

At this stage, they're still trying to help the driver to recover from dangerous conditions, with assists like Anti-lock Braking Systems and Electronic Stability Control.

4. Crash is unavoidable.

Now the goal is to minimize the damage with technology like Intelligent Brake Assist and Pre-Crash Seat Belt loading.

5. Crash

Now you hope to come out of it alive and maybe even uninjured with zone body construction and supplemental restraint-system airbags.

6. Post-crash

What's needed now is an automatic emergency call service.

Now let's look generically at the safety systems referred to and some additional ones. Remember, all the manufacturers have their own terminology or brand names for all this stuff so don't get confused by the names. You have to be able to understand what it actually does.

Early Driver Assistance Systems
Anti-lock Braking System

The first of the electronic safety technologies most of us experienced was ABS and it arrived as an expensive option in the 1980s. ABS keeps the wheels from locking up when you brake hard, to prevent uncontrolled skidding.

People thought they were buying it in order to stop faster. In fact, on gravel, or wet slippery roads, or snow-covered roads ABS can significantly increase braking distance. That's because ABS is making the brakes go on-off, on-off in milliseconds. The point of it is to improve vehicle control to let you steer around a problem, rather than slide into it.

Although I wonder how many people actually understand what it's good for, ABS is standard equipment now.

Electronic Stability Control

Anti-lock braking systems have now evolved into something else. ABS still prevents wheel-lock under braking, but it has been extended to also electronically control the front-to-rear brake bias and/or side-to-side traction. This is called Electronic Stability Control (ESC) and it too is standard equipment in all 2014 vehicles. ESC helps control your vehicle when you need to swerve or brake suddenly, to avoid an obstacle, by automatically braking one or more wheels for short periods of time and if necessary, reducing engine power.

In the United States, the Insurance Institute for Highway Safety found that ESC could help avoid 41% of single-vehicle collisions, while a study by the US National Highway Traffic Safety Administration shows that ESC could cut down the number of single-car collisions by 35%. ESC is a great safety feature because it keeps you from spinning out. You'll never know you have it until you need it.

Rear-View (Back up) Camera

The US National Highway Traffic Safety Administration will require automakers to install back-up cameras in all vehicles by May 2018.

Approximately 15,000 people are injured annually in backover accidents in the U.S. each year. Children younger than 5 account for 31% of the 210 people killed annually in these accidents, while people older than 70 account for 26%.

"We are committed to protecting the most vulnerable victims of backover accidents — our children and Seniors," said Transportation Secretary Anthony Foxx.

This idea has been debated for years; meanwhile the price of the cameras has come way down as several manufacturers are installing them as standard equipment. You can be sure the next step will be the elimination of side view mirrors and their replacement with cameras also – a change that would improve a vehicle's aerodynamics and thus fuel-efficiency.

Advanced Driver Assistance Systems

The acronym is ADAS and these are systems to help the driver in the driving process. Some simply warn the driver of an impending peril, while the "active" systems actually brake or steer the car for you. Many of these systems require Radar (RAdio Detection And Ranging) that uses radio waves to determine the range, direction, and speed of objects or Sonar (SOund Navigation And Ranging), which emits pulses of sound and listens for echoes to locate objects much the way dolphins and bats have for centuries.

Adaptive Cruise Control

ACC is cruise control that automatically adjusts the vehicle speed to maintain a safe distance from vehicles ahead. It also goes by the name of radar cruise control, for obvious reasons. It will hit the brakes for you to slow you down and bring your vehicle to a complete stop, if necessary. ACC technology is a key component of any self-driving cars.

Blind Spot Detection

This driver-assistance device senses cars coming up in your blind spot, behind or alongside you. If your turn signal is on, it alerts you not to change lanes. You're warned by a flashing light on the side view mirror and then a beep or maybe a seat or steering wheel vibration. If you're not planning to change lanes, because you haven't put the turn signal on, the warning light glows steadily but doesn't flash and there's no audible alert.

It can work off video sensors (cameras) and/or laser sensors and/or infrared sensors, as do the lane-keeping systems below.

Lane Departure Warning

LDW warns a driver when the vehicle begins to move out of its lane (unless a turn signal is on in that direction) with visual, audible, and/or vibration warnings.

Lane Keeping System

LKS warns the driver and if no action is taken, automatically takes steps to steer the vehicle back into its lane.

Collision Avoidance System

Also known as a pre-crash system or a forward-collision warning system, it uses radar and sometimes laser and camera sensors to detect an imminent crash. Once the detection of an imminent collision is made, these systems either provide a warning to the driver, or in an active system, take action autonomously by braking, steering or both, without any driver input.

Night Vision

A night vision system helps drivers see distant objects in darkness or poor weather, beyond the reach of the vehicle's headlights.

Driver Drowsiness Detection

It has various names; Ford calls it Driver Alert, Mercedes-Benz calls it Attention Assist. It is a system that monitors the driver's drowsiness level, based on his/her driving inputs and assesses whether the vehicle is being driven in a safe way. It issues a visual and audible alarm to tell the driver to take a break.

Survive the Crash

All the new vehicles on the road have vastly improved crash-worthiness and rollover safety standards. Safety cages built into vehicles diffuse impact energy in the passenger compartment and provide strong foundation structure. Crumple zones literally crumple up in a collision, absorbing the energy of the collision, diverting it from the passenger compartment and keeping the safety cage intact. Side impact, cross-car beams help channel energy during a collision. Multiple air bags help restrain the driver and front passenger, in moderate-to-severe front impacts.

The gold standard for overall safety ratings is the Five Star system created by the US National Highway Traffic Safety Administration (NHTSA). You can find their vehicle ratings at www.safercar.gov.

Background to Nissan Safety Technology

Nissan uses the term, Safety Shield, to describe a system that monitors 360-degrees around the car, for risks, offers warnings to the driver, and takes action to prevent an accident.

Nissan uses various forms of advanced sensors, including laser scanners and monitor-cameras, to take in the full 360-degree circle surrounding the vehicle; looking for obstacles, other vehicles and potential risks, as well as road signs and signals. That of course feeds into processing power and software that enables the car to react to the data the advanced sensors collect.

Let's have a chat with the man responsible for product planning for all Nissan and Infiniti vehicles throughout the Americas.

FEATURE INTERVIEW

With Pierre Loing, Vice President, Product Planning, Nissan Americas.

Vaughan

I think a lot of people don't order optional safety equipment because they don't understand it.

Loing

These types of features are not easy to explain standing still. But blind-spot warning or around-view monitor, or intelligent cruise control – when someone buys it and uses it, then it's the kind of feature that they want to keep. But if it was just described to them, a lot of people would say, 'Nah, I don't need it. I've driven all my life without it.' But when you get used to it, you're hooked.

Vaughan

I also know people who rely on it too much and get lazy about their driving.

Loing

We have to be careful. Once you give customers technology – they tend to trust technology so much that they don't pay a lot of attention anymore. I remember in the first days of ABS, in Germany, the insurance companies were giving rebates for vehicles equipped with ABS but later, they noticed that the rate of accidents with ABS was in fact higher. The customers could not understand ABS. They said, 'I had ABS and my car didn't stop.' Yes, it will help you stop but you are in a moving object weighing one and a half or two tonnes and it has speed, so you have to remain in control.

Vaughan

I had that experience myself. When I first got it, I went out and tested it; going straight on a snow-covered road and it did take longer to stop. But the point is, you can steer the car while you're stopping and hopefully steer around the problem. I didn't know that Day One.

Loing

We have said that we want to put an autonomous driving car on the road by the end of the decade. That doesn't mean the car should be driving itself without anybody paying attention.

Vaughan

People also need to understand that some safety systems give you a warning and some can step in and control the car. That's a big difference in the systems.

Loing

The goal is zero fatalities. Let's look at what's looking out ahead of the vehicle for you.

Intelligent Cruise Control uses radar and will adjust your speed when it gets within the set distance of the car in front.

Forward Collision Warning uses the same type of technology and will alert you when it detects that the distance between you and the car in front is becoming critical…beep beep beep…it is telling you to do something. Forward Collision Warning does not brake the car.

Forward Emergency Braking is basically the same system but it will stop the vehicle when it detects that if it doesn't stop the vehicle, it will be too late.

The step after that is the Predictive Forward Collision Warning, which is Nissan's distinct technological innovation. It is a mixture of camera looking at the vehicle in front of you, and radar to go under the vehicle in front of you, to determine what is happening two cars ahead. When the system detects potential risks, it signals the driver to decelerate. It gives the signal on the display, plus an audible warning, and also by tightening the seat belt.

Vaughan

If you're covering 360 degrees, what's checking the side of the car?

Loing

On the side, you have Blind Spot Warning. That's a technology that is widespread now. Depending on the vehicle, either the camera, or the camera and the sonar will tell you there's a vehicle in the angle where you can't see it. We put Blind Spot Warning in Rogue and even the Versa Note.

The next step is the Blind Spot Intervention, which will brake the wheels on the side opposite to where the unseen vehicle is and bring your car back into its lane.

Vaughan

What's looking behind you?

Loing

We have Rear View Monitor with camera at the back or Around View Monitor, when you rely on four cameras around the vehicle that you typically use when you park or manoeuvre at low speed.

Back-up Collision Intervention is two things. You have the moving object detection that is camera-based and that analyzes image by image. Typically, when you back up, it will beep when there is a moving object detected within the camera's scope.

Back-up Collision Intervention adds the braking function on top of it and that is camera and sonar-based as well. The predictive systems are the most complex because the vehicle has to do everything on its own. These new breakthroughs help detect and avoid a potential risk from an early stage, before the situation becomes critical.

Vaughan

What is the plan to roll these features out across the line-up?

Loing

What I have described is common in Infiniti and is available in Nissan. They are relatively expensive technologies because they rely on expensive equipment, so they are more popular on higher-end vehicles. Infiniti is more advanced, in terms of equipment, than Nissan. I would say there's 50 or 60% take rate on the advanced safety suite on the high-end vehicles. But we offer rear-view camera monitoring and other safety features even on our entry-level vehicles.

. . . .

Background to General Motors Safety Technology

General Motors focuses on safety – before, during, and after an accident. Here is the range of their available, not all standard, safety technologies.

Before Crash

All-Wheel Drive adjusts torque distribution within a fraction of a second and sends torque to the wheels with the best traction.

Anti-lock Braking System helps the driver maintain proper vehicle steering control during hard braking, even on slick surfaces.

Traction Control automatically applies brake pressure to appropriate wheels, to limit wheelspin and help re-establish traction.

Electronic Stability Control intervenes automatically, to help prevent lateral skids and restore steering control.

Proactive Roll Avoidance on most SUVs reduces the vehicle's tendency to roll over in a panic situation.

Xenon High Intensity Discharge Headlights improve visibility compared to conventional Halogen headlights.

Articulating Headlights automatically pivot to illuminate the area you're steering towards.

Magnetic Ride Control suspension employs sensors that read the road 1000 times a second, to automatically adjust the damping of each individual shock absorber.

Lane Departure Warning and Side Blind Zone Alert use a camera, mounted in the rear-view mirror, to read the lines on the road. Should the vehicle stray, the system alerts the driver via visible and audible cues.

During Crash

Seatbelt Pre-tensioners reduce slack that may exist in a seatbelt system at the moment of a frontal collision.

Front air bags help restrain the driver and front passenger in moderate-to-severe front impacts. Dual-depth units automatically adjust the deployment of the air bags, based on the severity of the collision, the seat position, and other factors.

Seat-mounted and head-curtain air bags provide additional protection in moderate-to-severe side impacts.

Safety Cage helps diffuse impact energy in the passenger compartment and provides strong foundation structure.

Crumple zones literally crumple up in a collision, absorbing the energy of the collision and diverting it from the passenger compartment.

Side-Impact Beams: Side-impact cross-car beams help channel energy during a collision.

After Crash

In a crash, when the air bags deploy, OnStar will automatically send a call for help with the exact location of the vehicle.

FEATURE INTERVIEW

With Brian Latouf, Director of Canadian Engineering, General Motors of Canada Ltd.

Vaughan

How does GM approach the field of driver- assistance technology?

Latouf

It's through building blocks of safety systems; some give you a warning and some can partially control the vehicle and assist in you in a driving event. That's an active system, not just a warning. We have several systems that assist the driver through warnings and messaging. We do that effectively but also through active engagement of the vehicle.

Vaughan

Let's talk about the active systems. What's available now?

Latouf

With Cadillac, we have things like forward-collision alert, side blind-zone alert, lane-departure warning, rear cross-traffic alert. On the XTS and ATS, we have a network of cameras, radar, and ultrasonic sensors, to help drivers avoid crashes by warning them of dangerous situations and even braking automatically, if the vehicle is at risk of crashing.

Vaughan

That's an active system. When would you get automatic braking?

Latouf

For example, if the vehicle is in stop-and-go traffic, the system will alert you if the lead vehicle slows unexpectedly and, if needed, brake your vehicle, to help prevent an impact or reduce impact speed.

We also have crash-imminent braking, so that with short-range and long-range radar systems, it knows if your vehicle is closing too quickly on the vehicle in front of you and it will actively brake.

And if the system senses a panic-braking situation, it automatically applies added brake force, to help slow the vehicle more quickly. This system uses radar and vision sensors.

Vaughan

What is the Safety Seat?

Latouf

It's Safety Seat Alert. It sets off seat vibrations on either the left or right side of the driver's seat, depending on the side of the impending problem. It works with other visual alerts, to focus the driver's attention to the direction of potential problems. Some drivers are annoyed by hearing beeping alerts. Although if they prefer, they can set the system to replace seat vibrations with beeps. It's a pretty effective system.

Vaughan

Does it matter how you warn them?

Latouf

It's about HMI – Human-Machine Interface. It is such an important part of how we engineer and design. That's why we talk about building blocks because as you introduce the technologies, you've got to see how they're accepted, how people react to them, how they use the systems and gain confidence in them. Is an audible and visual warning more effective than a vibration in a seat? How do you engage that driver when they're doing other things?

Vaughan

I notice the advanced active systems are on Cadillac but what about Chevy Cruze?

Latouf

The reality of some of these active systems is that you need to put sensors on the vehicles that see outwards – embedded sensors – and it gets very expensive to have cameras and radars. Plus these systems have to cross-talk. We call it sensor fusion.

If you're going to brake the vehicle, you have to have confidence that the sensor wasn't seeing a flying piece of paper or something that's not appropriate. You have to make the correct decision. So we have redundant systems in place and sensors there to confirm, and that adds additional cost.

If you're trying to bring to market a very cost-effective, sub-compact vehicle, it's very difficult to put all these technologies onto the product and be cost competitive. So we're trying to figure out lower-cost systems. That's part of the engineering effort. Can you do all this with just cameras, because cameras are fairly cheap, and not have to do all the radars?

Vaughan

So in some segments, this active technology isn't there yet?

Latouf

When you warn a driver, you don't need the confidence that you do when you actively brake the vehicle, or steer the vehicle. So a camera system alone can provide you with the knowledge to do a warning. So it's much easier to integrate a warning system into a Cruze or a Sonic than the active systems that actually brake and steer the vehicle. So we can offer that into the compact and sub-compact segments. We offer forward-collision alert and blind-zone alert and lane-departure warning and we package them as options.

Mercedes-Benz Driver-Assistance Systems

All the car companies are working on driver-assistance systems, with the aim of preventing accidents from happening or mitigating their consequences but Mercedes has been first to market with many of them.

Mercedes-Benz is a "premium" brand, in other words, expensive. It's no surprise therefore that Mercedes can be at the forefront of the introduction of many of the new technologies, simply because their customers can afford to purchase them. Having said that, Mercedes has been very fast at putting them into lower-priced models than the S-Class.

They're marketed under the banner of the Mercedes-Benz Integrated Safety Concept. Nissan defines six phases of driving situations. Mercedes covers the same ground, divided into four phases. They are worth looking at, along with the technology designed to help.

1. Safe every-day driving
2. Critical situations

3. During an accident

4. After an accident

1. Safe every-day driving

The majority of accidents start long before the actual collision; and they're mostly caused by concentration lapses, poor visibility, and hazards. Mercedes-Benz technology helps prevent everyday occurrences from becoming bad-day problems.

Passive Blind-Spot Assist

Indicators on the side mirrors light up when there's a vehicle in the blind spot, thus alerting the driver before he or she changes lanes, right into an adjacent car.

Passive Lane-Keeping Assist

Passive Lane-Keeping Assist identifies when the driver is drifting out of a lane unintentionally. The driver is warned by means of a vibration in the steering wheel.

Attention Assist

The system warns the driver visually and audibly, if it detects signs of failing attention and increasing weariness.

Brake Assist

Based on the speed with which the brake pedal is depressed, it can identify an emergency braking situation and then automatically build up full braking power to the slip threshold, so that steering control is maintained.

2. Critical situations

Bad conditions are a reality of driving and an extra set of eyes is never a bad thing; especially one that can anticipate accidents before they happen.

Electronic-Stability Program

In critical situations, an Electronic-Stability Program can help to stabilize the vehicle by applying a braking force to individual wheels and adjusting engine performance. The yaw-rate sensor continuously measures the vehicle movement around its vertical axis. As soon as the vehicle deviates from the ideal figures, the system intervenes by counteracting any swerving movements as soon as they occur.

Antilock Brakes

ABS helps to prevent the wheels from locking, in order to maintain their steering function.

3. During an accident

Airbags

The adaptive front airbags monitor the predicted severity of a collision and will deploy in two stages. To reduce the risk of injury in minor collisions, the airbag is only partially filled.

In lateral impacts that exceed a defined impact-threshold, the window curtain airbags are deployed on the impact side.

Driver's-knee airbags

If the crash sensors detect a collision of a threshold strength, the knee airbag is deployed on the driver's side to protect the legs during impact.

Pelvis airbags

If the crash sensors detect a relevant side collision, the pelvis airbag is deployed to provide protection for the pelvic region and hip.

Side airbags

The side airbags fitted as standard for the driver and front passenger provide side-body protection for occupants in the event of an impact.

Windowbags for driver and front passenger

In the event of an excessive side impact, the window airbags deploy to reduce the risk of a collision between the passenger's head and the side of the vehicle, or with objects penetrating the vehicle interior. The window airbag is triggered simultaneously with the side and pelvis airbags, on the side of impact.

4. After an accident

The engine is switched off automatically and the fuel supply is cut off.

Hazard-warning lamps and emergency interior-lighting are activated automatically, to prevent rear collisions and make it easier for rescue workers to find the vehicle.

Doors are automatically unlocked. Integrated crash joints between the wing and door are sped up, allowing rescue workers to open doors easily after a frontal collision.

The Self-Driving Mercedes

>Let's take a drive with the man who is in charge of all passenger car development for Mercedes-Benz world-wide, Prof. Dr. Thomas Weber; Member of the Board of Management of Daimler AG.

In spite of his powerful title, Weber is an engineer's engineer. He likes nothing better than going deep into the engineering details of the latest products and answers questions like he's defending a PhD thesis, rather than spitting out PR sound bites.

We took our drive as part of the global media launch of the new Mercedes S-Class. This is the mighty sedan that ferries around German chancellors, bank presidents, or anyone who can write a very large cheque.

The latest member of the $120,000-and up line is on the market now. It is a car that can drive itself – but is not allowed to. With Weber behind the wheel, we drove to a busy expressway.

I commented glibly, "You could make this car drive itself and sell it today, if it weren't for the liability lawyers."

He replied seriously, "This discussion you cannot have, independent of the legal framework. But our key message is yes. Autonomous driving will start with the new S-Class. All the hardware systems on board, for example, radar-based distronic1 systems, short, medium, and long-range radar and a stereo camera mounted above the windshield. With these two systems, we now are able to give the car the function of autonomous driving."

"But not now," said I.

Weber replied, "We equipped the S-Class for customers in Silicon Valley, China, and Europe who say they have terrible traffic from home to office and say it would be really helpful if somebody controls the situation for them. For example, now I am discussing with you and I can concentrate on you."

At this point, we're doing the speed limit in traffic and Weber takes his hands off the steering wheel and continues to look at me, not the road. The car stays in its lane while steering itself and following the car ahead at a consistent distance.

"You see, the car follows the car ahead of us. We are controlled by distronics and the stereo camera is checking to see that everything is okay. We call it Stop and Go Pilot. It's a comfort system. It assists you. The system checks critical situations and helps you. If necessary, the car stops automatically."

To make sure you don't get lazy and rely on the system too much while filing your nails or checking emails, the system gives you ten seconds-maximum hands free. A light on the dash flashes after a

---

1

couple of seconds, then a tone starts ringing, and if you still haven't taken the wheel it slows you right down.

"The idea is not to give the customer the feeling that they do not have to pay attention because that is not our philosophy. Nevertheless, you have a comfortable feeling that someone is behind the curtain helping you to manage the situation."

All the major manufacturers are working on autonomous driving systems with similar functionality. I have driven Volvos and Nissans with excellent capabilities. The ability of the stereo camera to see and process images of things rapidly approaching from the sides – whether a pedestrian or a moose – is particularly helpful. The system will hit the brakes if you don't and many a crash can be avoided.

The Mercedes system can also tell the difference between the pedestrian and the moose. If it's a pedestrian, as it hits the brakes, it sends a spotlight's highest beam at the person; to hopefully make him or her stop too. If it's a moose, deer, dog, or whatever it recognizes the shape and still hits the brakes but avoids the beam so as not to startle the animal, which might charge the light. It gets complicated.

"So whose fault is it if there is an accident?" I asked. "Who gets sued? The software, the radar, the stereo camera, or Mercedes-Benz?"

Replied Weber, "All these topics we have to clarify in detail with the regulators. It is definitely clear when it comes to these autonomous situations we have to integrate some additional checking systems so that we can show after an accident what really happened. An airplane uses a black box, which always checks the key figures."

So autonomous driving is here now, in a limited way. Now you can drive and be assisted by "someone behind the curtain," with a little black box recording everything that goes on. Will this prevent accidents? In my view –definitely yes.

CHAPTER 7

My Top Fifty Picks

One of the greatest frustrations about covering the automotive industry is the number of times I'm asked the simplistic question, "What's the best car?"

And I answer, "For what?"

The best car – and a better term is vehicle because you might want an SUV, which is classified as a light truck – is determined by matching your particular needs, tastes, driving habits, and budget to a product. Take your time, do your research, and really think about your choices. No one should be brand loyal anymore; you'll overlook too many great choices that way.

And remember this – the vehicle you buy must put a smile on your face every time you get into it. Get it wrong and you'll be cursed by "Buyer's Remorse," as long as you own it.

The following are not just the best vehicles for old people. These are, in my opinion, the best vehicles for everyone.

The automotive market is divided into segments, or classes, of vehicles. Some analysts divide it up so finely they come up with dozens of segments and sub-segments and sub-sub-segments.

I'm going to look at the market in terms of "only" ten segments and I think you'll find it useful if you approach the market this way.

I'm going to list them from the smallest vehicle to the largest.

The biggest segment in Canada and the U.S. year after year is full-size pickup trucks. I'm going to skip this segment because I don't know how many readers of this book are in the market for one of these big, powerful work trucks. Besides, truck buyers are so brand-loyal they wouldn't listen to my advice anyway.

I'll skip the hundred thousand-dollar sports cars too for similar reasons.

I think the most interesting and appropriate choices will be in Compact Cars, Compact SUVs and Luxury Compact Crossovers; those are the segments to which I'll pay the most attention.

So Many Choices

So what are our criteria? What should we be looking for in a new vehicle? The question that you must answer is, "Is this car right for me?"

I'll be evaluating them on the basis of having the best: Comfort and Convenience, Value, Safety Features and the new one, Driver-Assistance Technology.

Comfort and Convenience includes the ergonomic issues and gets to things like ease of entry and exit, comfortable seating, visibility, and adjustability (powered preferred) of seating, pedals, steering wheel, doors, trunks, mirrors etc.

Value is all about the total cost of ownership, including price, operating and maintenance costs, reliability, fuel economy, and resale value.

Safety Features include rear backup camera, front and rear sensors and warning systems, and overall safety rating.

Driver Assistance Technologies are the new camera and radar-controlled systems that see things you might not see, and steer and stop the vehicle, as well as provide active parallel park assistance.

Research, Research, Research

These will be little thumbnail sketches of selected vehicles, not in-depth analyses. They're intended to help you narrow down your choice; then you're ready to do some serious research on your own before you write the check.

Consumer Reports does a great job of evaluating new vehicles and their new-car buying guides are worth the money.

But there's also local pricing to research. Everybody likes buying things on sale and that includes cars and trucks. There are great deals out there but you have to work to find them. Do some research on the Internet and you'll never pay sticker price again.

All cars, CUVs and SUVs listed below are 2014 models. Here's my top fifty:

SUB COMPACT CARS

Don't rule out a sub-compact if you've never owned one – or haven't owned one recently. They are comfortable, nimble, and well suited to safe urban driving. Some people are stuck in the belief that these are still just cheap econo-boxes. Nothing could be further from the truth.

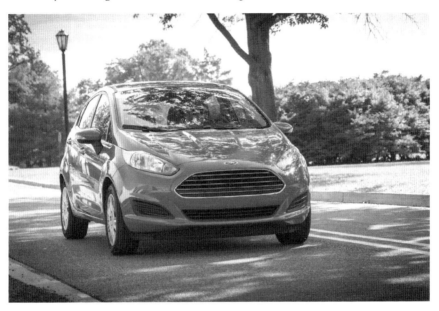

FORD FIESTA – Small cars are fun to drive and in the Fiesta, with its nimble handling and great feel for the road, you'll be smiling too. It was restyled for 2014, which made a huge improvement in looks. A four-cylinder engine is perfectly adequate but it won't pin you back with acceleration. A five-speed manual transmission is standard and a six-speed automated manual transmission is optional.

Don't opt for the sporty ST model – too noisy and rough riding. Ford learned to build small cars this good in Europe where drivers really appreciate them. You will too when you drive it and see the reasonable price tag.

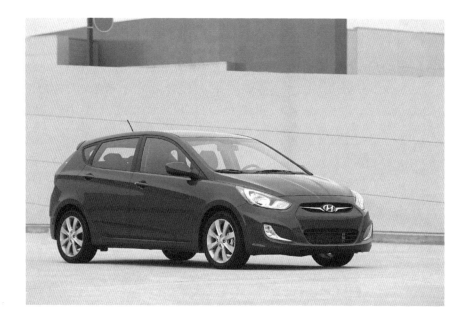

HYUNDAI ACCENT – This is the fourth-generation of the Accent sedan and they just keep getting better. There's more room in it than you think, and it looks more premium than the price would lead you to believe. As usual, I like the hatchback version better than the sedan. The bright colors and its high-power audio appeal to the kids – but why should they have all the fun?

Like its stablemate the Kia Rio, Accent has an amazing 10-year/100,000-mile power train warranty. You really can't beat it for the price but if you have any trouble bending down low, you might find anything in this class a bit of a struggle to get in and out of.

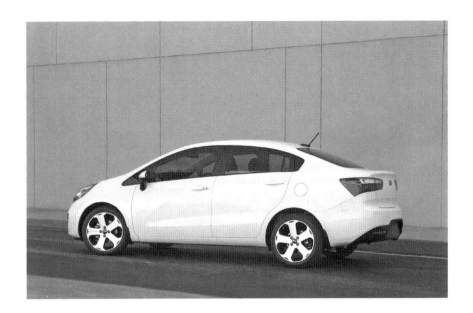

KIA RIO – Rio is just as good as Accent but with different styling and different dealers. You'll be surprised at how well it rides and how good the interior looks. Don't be reluctant to drive it on the highway because the 138 horsepower engine has plenty of power for both city and highway driving.

There's plenty of room in the front and even the back seats are totally usable for two adults. Optional features include a rear-view camera, although visibility in all directions is good. You'll be impressed with the 10-year/100,000-mile power train warranty. It even comes as a hatchback version with the Rio%, which is the one I'd choose.

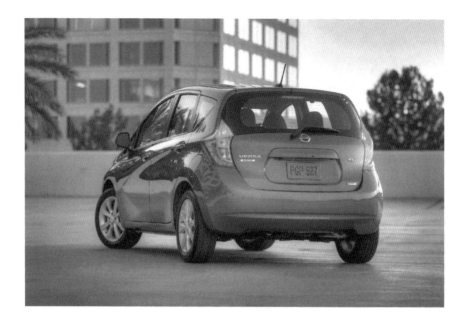

NISSAN VERSA NOTE – The bargain-basement price catches your eye first and if you're looking for a little car to get around town, then why not save some money? The Versa's interior is extremely basic but roomy. Four adults can ride in reasonable comfort. All the gauges are clear and legible and the controls are large and logically-placed.

The hatchback adds functionality and cargo space is generous. You can add features like keyless access, push-button start and a rear-view camera. It's slow but it hardly burns fuel at all. For basic, no-frills transportation you've got yourself a deal.

COMPACT CARS

Even if you have driven full-size sedans for years, it's time to consider a "compact" car. First, they're bigger than you think and second, they are just as comfortable quiet and safe as the big stuff, yet are more economical and easier to drive.

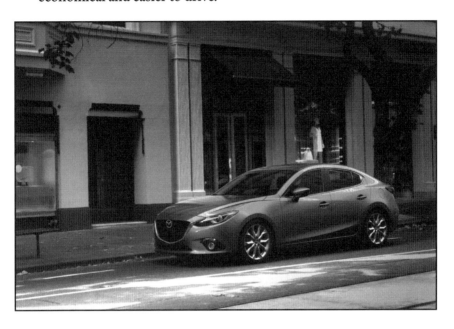

MAZDA3 – Everything about it makes it feel like a more expensive car. Mazda3 has won numerous awards as the best compact on the market. I prefer the 5-door (hatchback) over the sedan, in both appearance and practicality. It comes standard with an all-new, four-cylinder engine and six-speed manual transmission.

Available safety and driver-assistance features include lane-departure warning, forward-collision warning, adaptive cruise control, a rear-view camera, and blind-spot monitoring. If all you want is a soft ride, then this one isn't for you. The Mazda3 is sporty and fun to drive, yet quite comfortable. Make sure you can get in and out of its low profile with ease and that the seats are to your liking. A top pick.

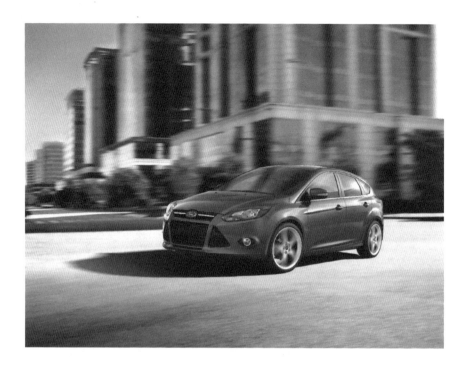

FORD FOCUS – You'll enjoy driving a Focus; you get precise steering, great cornering, and a comfortable ride. Get the 5-door not the sedan, for both looks and cargo room. Focus comes with standard front seat-mounted, side airbags as well as front and rear side-curtain airbags. Options include rear-parking sensors, a backup camera, and keyless entry and ignition.

Focus is powered by an efficient, but not overwhelming, four-cylinder engine and a six-speed automatic is available. I don't recommend the Focus ST with powerful turbocharged engine – too noisy, too stiff. With its upscale interior, comfortable seats, plenty of roominess, and excellent fuel economy, the Focus is the best compact cat Ford has ever built.

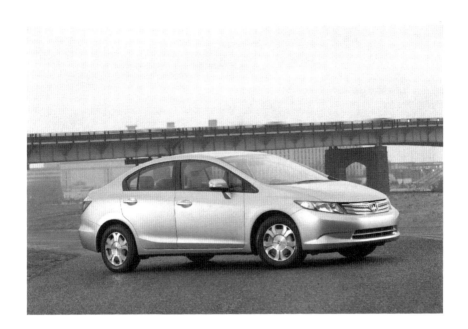

HONDA CIVIC – The made-in-Canada Civic has been the bestselling car in Canada for 16 years in a row. Who can argue with Civic's smooth power train, faultless reliability, and strong resale value? The 2014 model has available a continuously variable transmission (CVT) that is very smooth and helps deliver the best fuel economy in the segment.

In the past, the Civic interior was pretty bleak but now there's a mix of high-quality plastics and soft-touch surfaces that make it more upscale. Options include a multi-angle, rear-view camera and a blind-spot warning indicator. Honda owners are very loyal and the new Civic is easily enough to keep them attached.

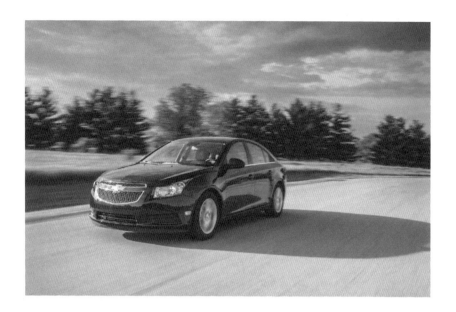

CHEVROLET CRUZE – The Cruze feels and drives like a bigger car. It is solid and quiet with a nice roomy interior. There are probably too many models to choose from – no less than six trim levels, three four-cylinder engines and even a diesel Cruze. The base four-cylinder engine is adequate in town and for highway cruising (not cruzing). I like the styling, the nimble handling, and the comfortable ride.

Standard features include 10 air bags, remote keyless entry and a tilt and telescopic steering wheel. Available features include a rear-view camera, rear-park assist, rear cross-traffic alert, and blind-spot monitoring. Cruze is a good car all around and GM's best compact ever.

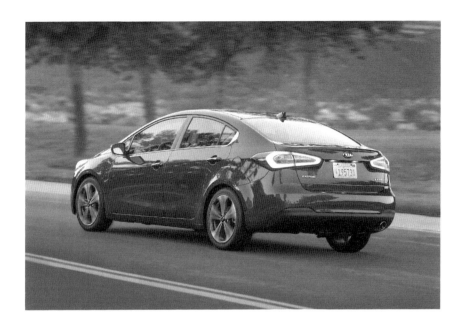

KIA FORTE – The new Forte is significantly improved over the previous model, as is the case with the entire Kia lineup. Build quality and overall refinement shows in the quietness of this car; at highway speed it's as quiet as many luxury cars. Forte is comfortable and has a spacious interior and lots of cargo space, especially with the 5-door – which is the best looking one too.

Kia used to be sold on their low price. Now the price is competitive but Forte still appeals for available features that most compacts don't offer, such as heated rear seats, fancy climate and infotainment systems, and a backup camera. The Kia Forte comes standard with a 1.8-liter four-cylinder engine, which works well with an optional six-speed automatic transmission.

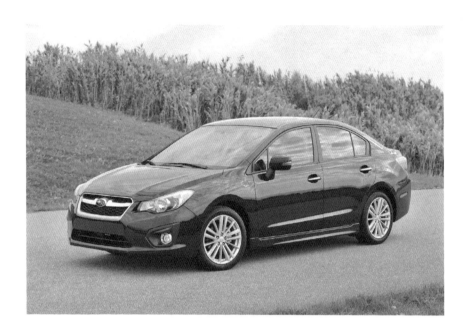

SUBARU IMPREZA – If you choose a Subaru, it's for the standard all-wheel drive and Impreza delivers it at the lowest price in the line-up. It's good value for the money but if you don't need all-wheel drive, you can find similar front-drive compacts with better fuel economy and a lower price.

Its base four-cylinder engine offers adequate power around town but you might wish it had a bit more power on the highway. A five-speed manual transmission is standard and a continuously variable transmission (CVT) is optional. The CVT helps with fuel economy. As usual, I like the hatchback better than the sedan. If you have to have AWD in your compact – look no further.

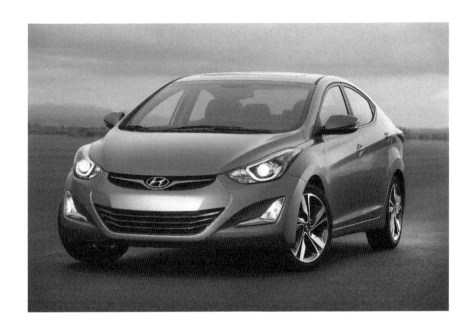

HYUNDAI ELANTRA – With a few upgrades for 2014, Elantra keeps on pleasing customers for value, fuel economy, interior quality, and warranty. It comes with a standard 1.8-liter, four-cylinder and a six-speed manual transmission, although a six-speed automatic is available.

Elantra is comfortable and fairly responsive but not what you would call sporty. It's been a hit, in part, because of its "swoopy" design – it's very striking but you might also be striking your head when you get into the back seat. It's impressive for safety; as it was awarded an IIHS Top Safety pick award and 5-star Overall Crash Safety Rating. I like the 4-wheel disc brakes on every model.

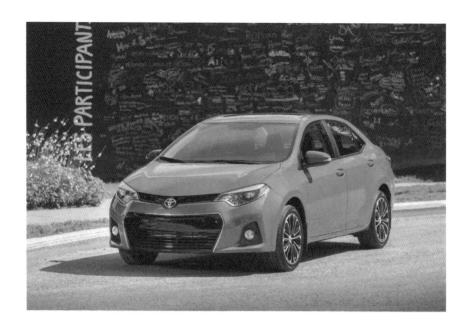

TOYOTA COROLLA – Corolla is a reliable commuter car that's easy, but not interesting, to drive. For 2014, Corolla has a rather old power train of a four-cylinder engine and an optional four-speed automatic transmission. It's slow to accelerate, especially with four people aboard.

The greatest difference in the new Corolla is a larger interior. It feels as large inside as the Camry – your back seat passengers will like this – but at a lower price. The cabin is mostly outfitted with hard, utilitarian plastics but it is roomy. A rear-view camera, cruise control, and keyless entry are options.

COMPACT CUVs

This is rapidly becoming the largest segment in the automotive marketplace. More people than ever are moving from cars to crossovers. They used to be called SUVs (Sport Utility Vehicles) when they were bigger and built on truck frames.

But now, the smaller versions are known as Crossover Utility Vehicles (CUVs) because they have "crossed over" from car platforms. Cars have unitized bodies and are not built on frames, making the vehicles lighter and better to drive. You have more than twenty choices in this popular segment; I'll try to help you narrow it down.

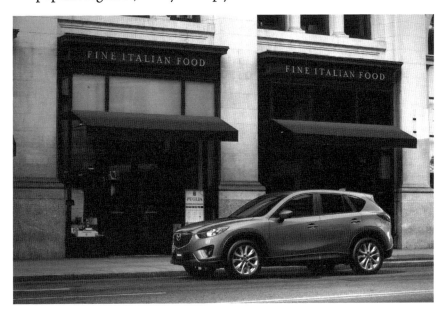

MAZDA CX5 – This is my favourite in the segment. Its excellent handling and precise steering make the CX-5 a pleasure to drive, while you enjoy excellent fuel economy. It's not the most powerful CUV by any means but the standard four-cylinder engine is perfectly adequate.

The interior is not plush but there's plenty of room inside and the controls are easy to reach and use. Standard features include keyless entry, push-button start, and steering wheel-mounted cruise and audio controls but you'll pay more for important options like a backup camera and a blind-spot monitoring system. If you enjoy driving and expect your vehicle to be more than a transportation appliance, then you have to check out the Mazda CX-5.

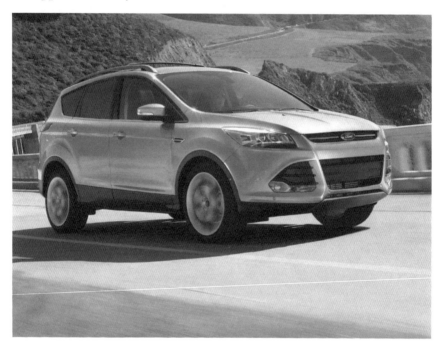

FORD ESCAPE – The Escape is built on the same platform as the Ford Focus, which makes it drive like a comfortable car – not a small truck. The base level, four-cylinder engine is adequate although there are other more expensive engine choices, along with the usual, six-speed automatic. The cabin is high quality and comfortable.

The Escape comes with a long list of standard features, including a backup camera and options like a motion-activated lift gate. You will either love or hate the often-frustrating MyFord Touch infotainment system, which you can control with voice commands. Do not buy it in this or any other Ford vehicle until you try it out and decide whether you like it. The touch screen in the center stack can be difficult to reach and the whole system can be a bit temperamental.

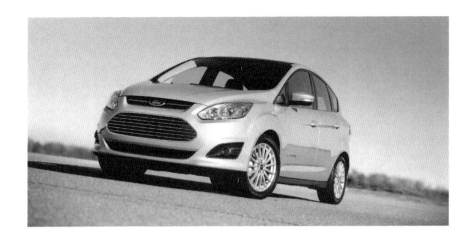

FORD C-Max – I haven't set aside a separate segment for hybrids because they are still only about 1% of total sales but I am recommending this one. The C-Max is also based on the Focus platform but in this case, it is a fun-to-drive hybrid with lots of passenger space. It has a four-cylinder gasoline engine, along with an electric motor. It can travel on electric power alone until the battery runs down, then the gasoline engine kicks in so quietly you hardly know it's on.

It's the same idea as the well-known Toyota Prius but the C-Max is a much more refined car. It has a great interior, although there isn't a huge amount of cargo space. Again, be sure you like the MyFord Touch system before you buy it and also check out the active park-assist, which helps steer the car into a parallel spot. It really works.

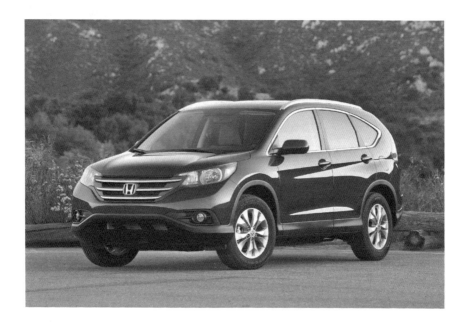

HONDA CR-V – The made-in-Canada CR-V has loyal repeat customers because of its excellent reliability. It has an efficient, four-cylinder engine and a standard, five-speed automatic transmission. The roomy interior gives a comfortable ride and the car handles well. Front-wheel drive is standard and all-wheel drive is optional. Even the base model CR-V has a standard backup camera.

It's not the most stylish vehicle in this very crowded segment but it stands out for its long-term quality scores and its high retained value. The CR-V was last redesigned in 2012 and is mostly unchanged for 2014 simply because they got it right the first time.

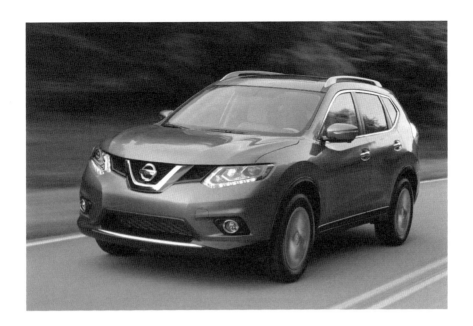

NISSAN ROUGE – Some markets are continuing to sell the 2013 Rogue at a slightly discounted price. That is not the one to buy. Rogue was redesigned for 2014 and it became a much-improved CUV. It's not sporty, in fact it's pretty soft from a driving performance point of view but it's a good soft. It has the most comfortable seats in the segment and with advanced stability control, it holds the road very well.

It could use a bit more power to work with its continuously variable transmission (CVT). Some people don't like CVTs but this is a good one and it helps deliver excellent fuel economy. Rogue comes standard with a rear-view camera but you'll pay more for Nissan's Around View monitor, which combines images from four cameras to give you a total view around the vehicle. This is a good safety feature and is terrific for parking,

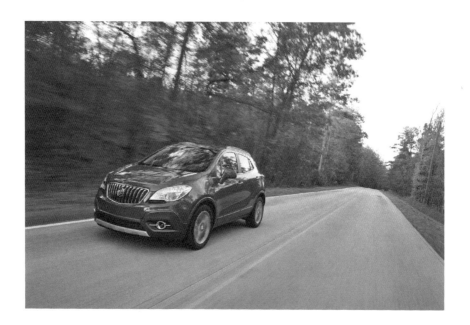

BUICK ENCORE – If you're used to Buicks being big old boats you're in for a surprise with the smallest Buick of all. The Encore is a tidy little CUV, featuring a turbocharged, four-cylinder engine and a six-speed automatic to deliver excellent fuel economy. The stylish cabin is trimmed with inexpensive-looking, soft-touch materials and Encore's front seats are comfortable and spacious.

You're paying a premium price for a Buick and the Encore does come with a long list of standard equipment, including a backup camera; but you should pay the extra for optional blind-spot monitoring with rear cross-traffic alert, forward collision, and lane-departure warning systems. It doesn't have overpowering performance but it handles well, delivering a comfortable ride. A good city car with a touch of luxury.

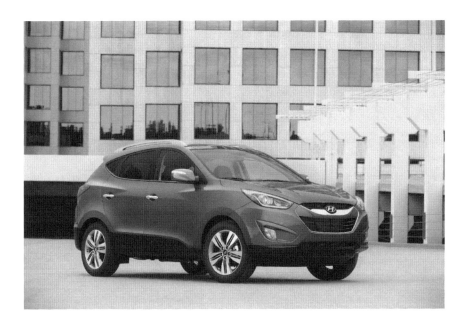

HYUNDAI TUCSON – Hyundai has served up a pleasant compact crossover at a reasonable price. Its manageable size makes it an interesting alternative to larger CUVs. It has a modern, four-cylinder engine and a six-speed automatic transmission – for good fuel economy rather than wild acceleration.

Its agility and small size lets it get in and out of tight spaces. The interior is of good quality and the layout is functional, with nice big gauges and controls. You have to be impressed with its 10-year/100,000-mile power train warranty.

MID-SIZE CUVs

The Mid-Size segment is a step up in size from the very popular Compact Crossover Utility Vehicles. If you're doing weekend trips to country or cottage and need a little more cargo room, you'll find great value in this category.

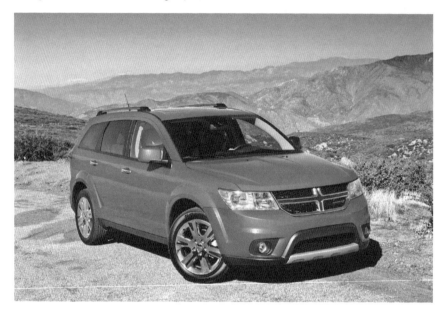

DODGE JOURNEY – Journey is a mid-size, seven-passenger crossover that's well worth considering for its versatile interior and affordable price. Make sure to choose the smooth and powerful V6 option over the lacklustre four-banger. The convenient interior with soft-touch materials is its strength. You get integrated child booster seats in the second row, and storage spaces in the rear floor and under the front passenger's seat.

The optional third row only has space for small children. All Wheel Drive is available along with useful options like rear-view camera and a parking assistance system.

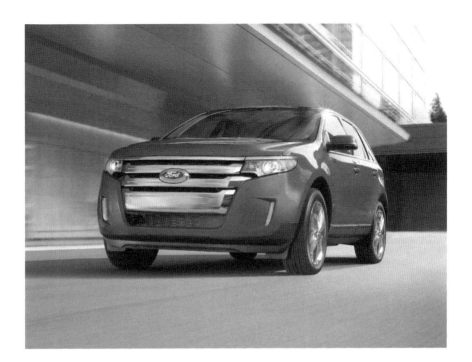

FORD EDGE – The Edge seats five comfortably for the long haul, along with lots of cargo space; in fact the interior seems like it comes from the luxury segment. There's plenty of choice in models and engines but avoid the expensive Sport because it rides too hard.

Optional safety features you want include adaptive cruise control and forward-collision warning. Be sure you try out the Ford SYNC system to make sure you like it. Overall, Edge is a trendy-looking, nice driving, and very functional mid-size crossover.

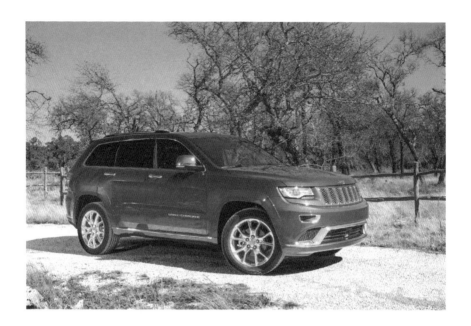

JEEP GRAND CHEROKEE – This is the best Jeep I have ever driven. The Grand Cherokee seats five and comes standard with rear-wheel drive but choose one of the all-wheel drive options because it really wouldn't be a Jeep if it were not fully off-road capable. There are a ridiculous number of models and trim levels and it will take you two weeks of research to find the one you like best.

When you do, you'll get a superb interior for comfortable cruising as well as off-road adventure. An eight-speed automatic transmission is standard on all Grand Cherokee models. It's fine for luxury options although it is quite short of the driver-assistance tech found in some competitors like the Ford Edge.

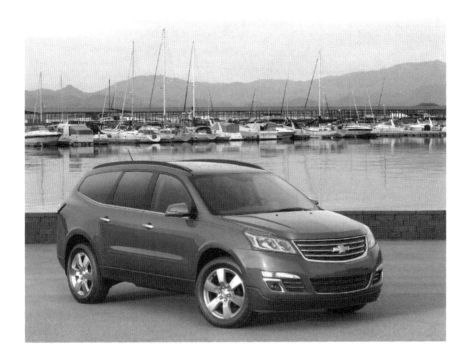

CHEVROLET TRAVERSE – The cabin is one of the most spacious in the class, as is the cargo space. There is seating for up to eight people, including the third row, which is best left to kids. Traverse is powered by a V6 engine along with a six-speed automatic. A rear-view camera is standard, while optional features include forward-collision alert and lane-departure warning.

It really is its enormous and functional cabin that impresses people, along with a comfortable ride and surprisingly nimble handling. It's a good alternative to a big, full-size SUV.

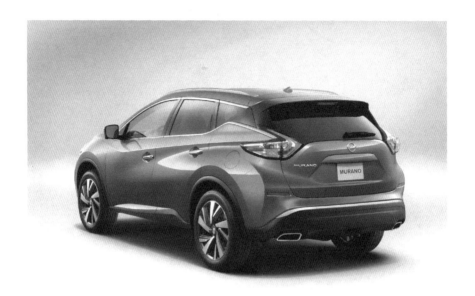

NISSAN MURANO – Murano has an interior that looks like it came out of a luxury SUV. The front seats are extremely comfortable, while giving a great view of the road. It has a V6 engine and continuously variable transmission (CVT), which is good for fuel economy once you get used to it. A rear-view camera is standard.

Front-wheel drive is standard but all-wheel drive is available. So is a convertible model…of all things. Murano is a quiet, comfortable, and refined midsize crossover, which stands out from others for its stylish design.

MID-SIZE CARS

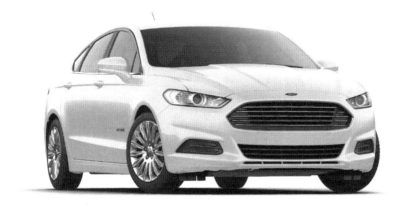

FORD FUSION – A few years ago, nobody would have believed that Ford could successfully compete in the mid-size range against the champs; Toyota Camry and Honda Accord. Ford has done so. Fusion with its pleasing styling, beautiful interior, and superior driving manners is a winner. Four different four-cylinder engines are offered, three are turbocharged, and a six-speed automatic is standard.

Also standard is the voice-controlled Sync with MyFord – check this out to see if you like it before you buy. Important options are adaptive cruise control with forward-collision warning, active park-assist, a rear-view camera, back-up sensors, rain-sensing wipers, blind-spot monitoring, and a lane-keeping alert system. There's also a hybrid version, which is better than Toyota's.

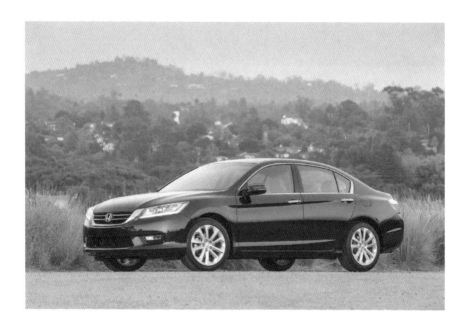

HONDA ACCORD – Accord gives you a handsome, spacious interior, good fuel economy, and better handling than most mid-size rivals. The standard four-cylinder engine is just fine, although a V6 is available. There's an optional continuously variable transmission (CVT) offered and it is probably the best one I've driven.

There is a standard rear-view camera and optional safety equipment includes adaptive cruise control, forward- collision warning and a blind-spot camera on the passenger-side mirror. There is now a hybrid Accord offered and it too is better than Toyota's. The previous Accord was a little dull – this one makes up for it.

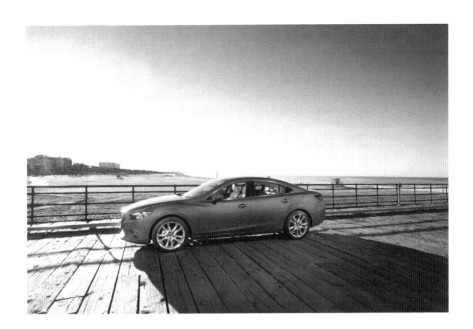

MAZDA6 – This is the fun-to-drive car of the mid-size class. It's all-new with dramatic exterior styling and a large, upscale interior. Mazda6 has a four-cylinder engine with a six-speed manual or automatic transmission. A V6 engine is no longer offered because it's not needed with the peppy, extremely fuel-efficient four.

Important safety features are optional, including a blind-spot monitoring system, a lane-departure warning system, forward obstruction warning and a rear cross-traffic alert system. This is the mid-size with some charisma – but that's a personal judgement. See it for yourself.

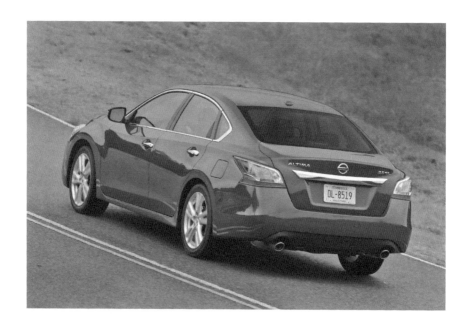

NISSAN ALTIMA – Nissan tells you they benchmarked the Audi A4 and BMW 3 Series when they designed the Altima and it shows. Excellent driving dynamics anda strong, four-cylinder engine with impressive fuel economy make this an athletic mid-size car. An optional six-cylinder engine is available but not necessary. All Altimas have a continuously variable transmission that operates quite smoothly.

You will probably love the comfort of the seats – the best in the class I think – although important safety equipment is only available as options, including blind-spot warning, lane-departure warning and moving-object detection. Altima sells very well in this highly completive segment for good reason.

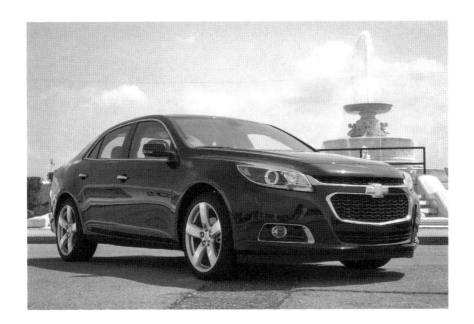

CHEVROLET MALIBU – It's getting a bit old now, although cosmetically improved but when it first came out several years ago, I called the Malibu the best sedan GM had ever built. Malibu comes with a four-cylinder engine and a six-speed automatic transmission that work well together. The suspension has been reworked and it's even smoother now. What stays the same is its quietness – it is almost serene inside even at highway speeds.

You pay extra for safety options including a rear-view camera, forward-collision alert, blind-spot warning and lane- departure warning. Not the most exciting car in the class but if you're a Chevy person you won't be disappointed.

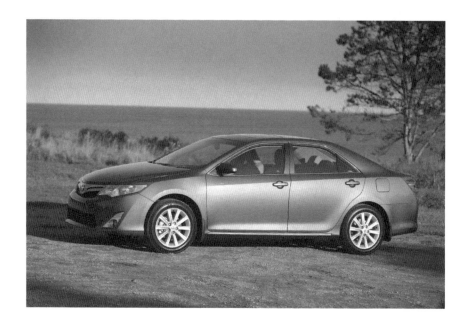

TOYOTA CAMRY – Its history of dependability might be its best selling point, along with its soft ride, good fuel economy and spacious interior. Camry's strong resale value adds to its reputation. It comes with a standard four-cylinder engine with a six-speed automatic transmission. A V6 is available though even that doesn't make it sporty but it delivers decent handling and a smooth and comfortable ride.

Safety features including blind-spot monitoring and cross-traffic alert are available as options. This latest edition of Camry is significantly improved yet it is the reputation for long-term value that keeps the Camry selling well.

MINIVANS

Don't be embarrassed to be seen in a minivan – they make perfect sense for people who have passengers and stuff to move about. They have been around for thirty years now and I predict they have another thirty ahead when the younger generations start having kids.

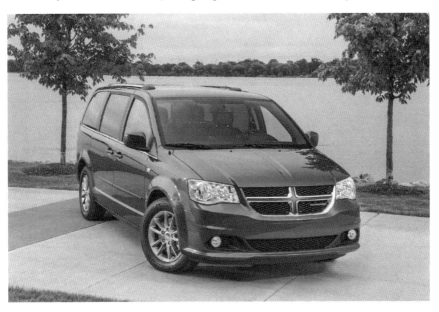

DODGE GRAND CARAVAN – It's not the most sophisticated minivan in the market but you cannot find better value than the made-in-Canada Dodge Caravan. It has a handsome and versatile interior, along with features including remote keyless entry. The optional features make this vehicle more user-friendly and they include power-sliding doors, blind-spot monitoring, and a rear-view camera. It puts the price up but it's worth it.

If you're a grandparent who needs to haul people and cargo and you don't want to blow the budget, then the Dodge Grand Caravan should top your list.

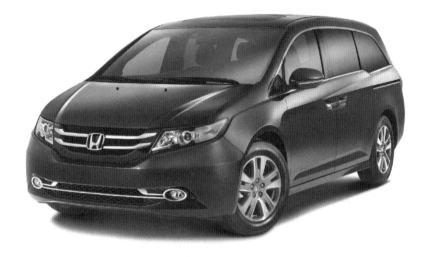

HONDA ODYSSEY – Odyssey is the best of minivans for quality, safety, and ride but it's also the most expensive. The Odyssey has a comfortable ride and responsive handling to go along with a spacious interior with comfortable seating in all three rows.

Standard features include power-adjustable front seats, an 8-inch color display, a rear-view camera, and remote keyless entry. You pay extra for worthwhile features like blind-spot monitoring, forward-collision warning, lane- departure warning, power sliding doors, a power tailgate, front and rear parking sensors, a rear-seat entertainment system, and navigation. It's the gold standard for people movers if you have the budget.

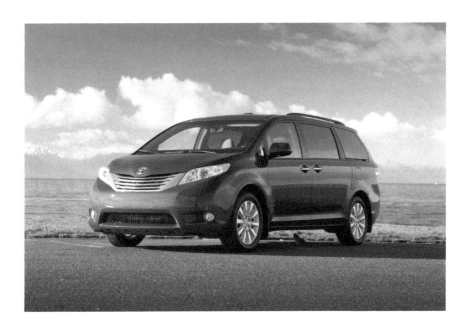

TOYOTA SIENNA – Sienna makes the list because it is reliable and safe and the only minivan that offers All Wheel Drive. It has a roomy interior although with a bit too much hard plastic but the three rows of seats are comfortable. It has a more powerful engine than the Odyssey.

Optional features include a rear-view camera, power-sliding rear doors, a power lift gate and blind-spot monitoring. With a wide range of models to choose from and strong resale value, Sienna is a popular choice.

LUXURY MID-SIZE CARS

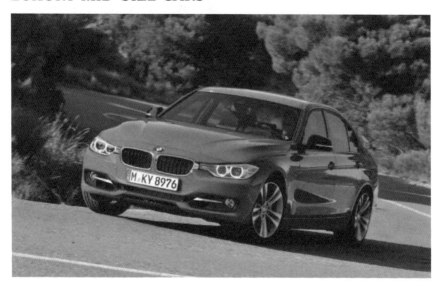

BMW 3-SERIES – The 3 Series is BMW's most important car and the best representative of BMW values. It's available now in three body styles with a turbocharged four-cylinder engine as standard, to go along with the famous inline six. You have the choice of a six-speed manual or eight-speed automatic transmission. It always has a superb interior to go along with sporty handling and a satisfying driving experience.

Safety features, available at extra cost, include a rear-view camera, side and top-view cameras, parking sensors, active cruise control, navigation, blind-spot detection, a head-up display and lane-departure warning. The 3 Series has set the standard for years but competitors are catching up.

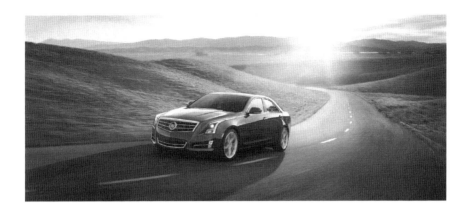

CADILLAC ATS – Cadillac has been obsessed with building a car to run with the best German sport sedans and ATS gets them there. The base engine is a normally aspirated four-cylinder but many buyers step up to the optional, turbocharged four-cylinder engine or the V6. ATS is a Caddy with balanced handling and a firm, comfortable ride. ATS is a North American sports sedan with a distinctly Cadillac look.

The interior is modern looking with high-quality materials but they might have gone too far with the optional CUE infotainment system, which has touch-sensitive controls that don't work very well. Options, besides CUE, which I would skip, include a rear-view camera, blind-zone alert, lane-departure warning, forward-collision alert and adaptive cruise control.

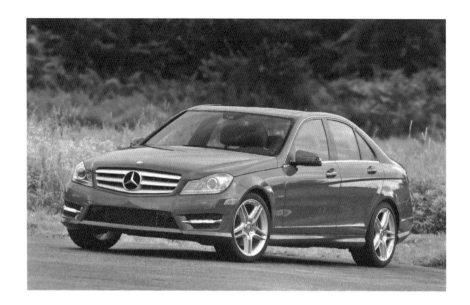

MERCEDES-BENZ C-CLASS – The 2014 C-Class has a handsome interior and is a pleasure to drive – but if you're thinking about buying one, you should wait until next year. The 2015 C-Class might be the one that gives BMW 3 Series a run for the money.

In 2015, the new C-Class drops 220 pounds from a lighter, stiffer body structure and adds many of the new safety technologies to the more expensive E-Class and S-Class, including a forward-collision warning system that can stop the car from speeds of up to 124 mph. Options include lane-keeping assist, adaptive cruise control, and active parking, as well as a surround-view camera.

But in the meantime, there should be some great deals on the 2014 C-Class, which is after all a safe, reliable, and classy car respected around the world.

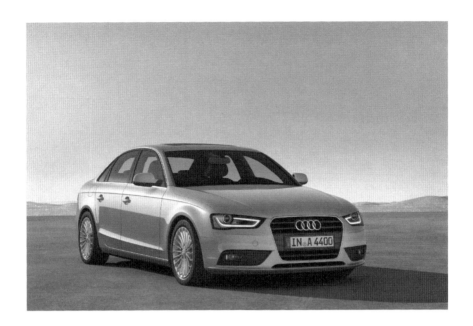

AUDI A4 – Audi sales have grown year after year by offering an upscale interior, comfortable ride and athletic performance. The 2014 Audi A4 base model comes with a turbocharged 2.0-liter four-cylinder engine. A continuously variable transmission (CVT) and front-wheel drive are standard, but most buyers seem to opt for the Quattro all-wheel drive system with either a six-speed manual or eight-speed automatic transmission.

The A4 received its last full redesign for the 2009 model year and has seen minor updates since then so it's getting a little old. An all-new A4 should be coming soon, which means some good deals on the current one should be available on this very pleasing car.

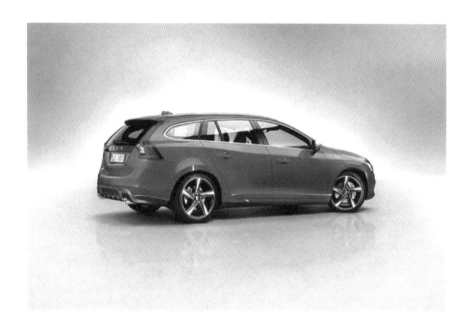

VOLVO V60 – Here's a great wagon in a sea of sedans. Volvo introduced its first wagon 60 years ago, and the V60 gets them back in the game. The V60 is a wagon with a bold new look but its clean lines remind you of the trusty Volvo station wagons of the past.

Volvo still tries to make their interiors look like high-end Swedish furniture and in that, the V60 succeeds. Under the hood is an all-new transverse, 2.0-liter inline-4 direct–injection gasoline engine. The V60 has standard City Safety, which prevents or mitigates slow-moving collisions with smart automatic braking. Optional is Pedestrian & Cyclist Detection, which with full auto brake can automatically stop you at speeds up to 31 mph if a person steps or swerves suddenly into your lane.

LUXURY COMPACT CROSSOVERS

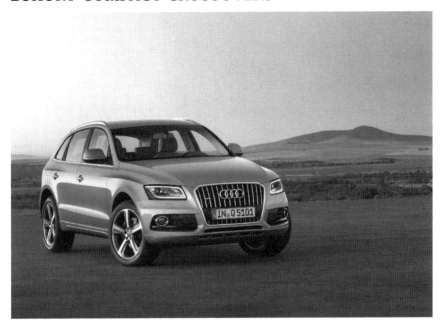

AUDI Q5 – Audi's 5-passenger luxury SUV has standard quattro all-wheel drive along with a premium interior and great driving dynamics. Q5 has a standard, turbocharged 2.0-liter four-cylinder engine and an eight-speed automatic, which delivers both performance and good fuel economy.

Audi is known for attractive interiors and excellent build quality. Seats are comfortable and roomy and provide excellent outward visibility. Options include adaptive cruise control, a rear-view camera, parking sensors, and a blind-spot monitoring system. Q5 had a facelift and some interior updates for 2014 but hasn't been fully redesigned since 2009. You might want to wait for the all-new and smaller Q3, which is arriving this year.

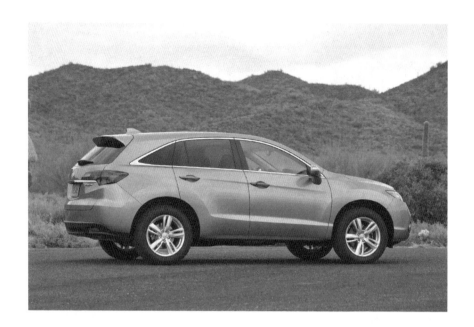

ACURA RDX – Restyled, re-engineered, and well priced, the RDX competes strongly in this segment. It has a strong, fuel-efficient V6, and a six-speed automatic transmission. It has standard front-wheel drive and all-wheel drive is optional. The cabin is both attractive and functional and this new edition rides much more comfortably than previously. It has a decent amount of cargo space and the low cargo floor makes it easy to load.

RDX has less advanced safety technology than others in the segment but it does have a rear-view camera. That's one of the ways they've kept the price down, which along with Acura's good record on long-term ownership costs, makes the RDX a good value.

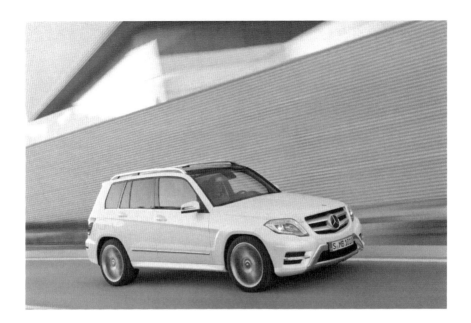

MERCEDES-BENZ GLK – The distinctive looking GLK-Class has seating for five but it's tight. However, the GLK comes standard with all-wheel drive and is powered by a turbo diesel 2.1-liter four-cylinder engine, which is a gem. Paired with a seven-speed automatic transmission, you have an extremely smooth and efficient power train.

It drives responsively for an SUV and while the interior isn't as roomy as some, it is a thing of beauty. All Mercedes have ample advanced safety equipment but the reason to buy the GLK is to get that great little diesel engine in a luxury crossover.

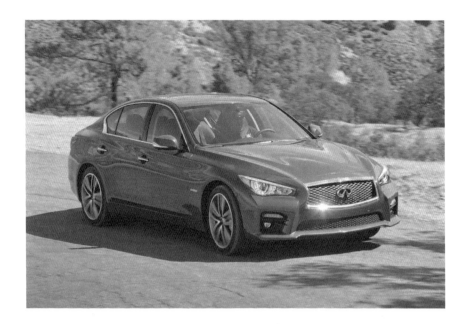

INFINITI Q50 – The Infiniti Q50 is an all-new model for 2014 with a powerful V6 engine and a refined, high-tech interior. A seven-speed automatic transmission is standard. The Q50's best feature might be the interior, which is well-built with premium materials including aluminum or wood trim.

The Q50 comes with standard features including a backup camera and optional safety features include blind-spot warning, forward-collision warning and lane-departure warning systems. Infiniti is trying hard to reinvent itself in order to catch up to the German premium brands. Progress is being made.

LUXURY SUVS

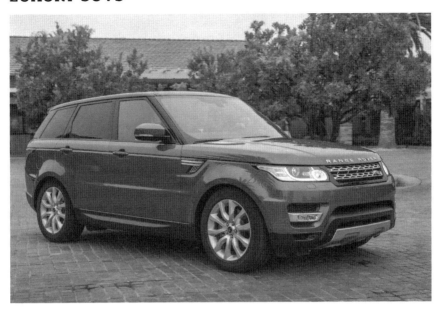

LAND ROVER RANGE ROVER SPORT –The Sport seats five; an optional third row adds two kids. Full-time four-wheel drive and a supercharged 3.0-liter V6 engine are standard. The Range Rover Sport was fully redesigned for 2014 with extensive use of aluminum, which succeeded in reducing 800 pounds of weight from the previous version, making it agile and quick. An eight-speed automatic transmission is standard.

The interior is first class. The ride on-road is comfortable and off-road it is amazing. Range Rover remains as distinct and exclusive as ever and as expensive as ever – but what an excellent, luxury midsize SUV.

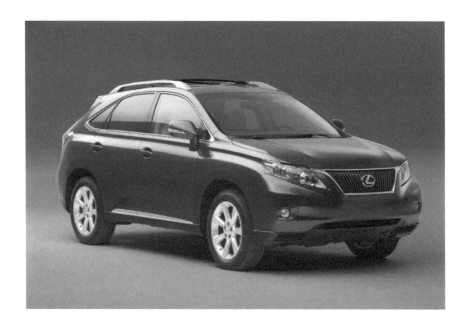

LEXUS RX 350 – Lexus RX has been money in the bank for Toyota since it was first introduced in 1998. It was one of the earliest luxury crossovers in the market and has remained one of the best. The RX exterior has become more stylish, in an aggressive way, and it delivers a soft, comfortable ride, especially for a SUV.

A 3.5L V6 engine and all-wheel drive is standard equipment in Canada and optional in the U.S. RX 350 offers a combination of luxury and practicality in a vehicle famous for its outstanding reliability. The current model is the 3rd generation and first went on sale in 2009. An all-new one is expected for 2015.

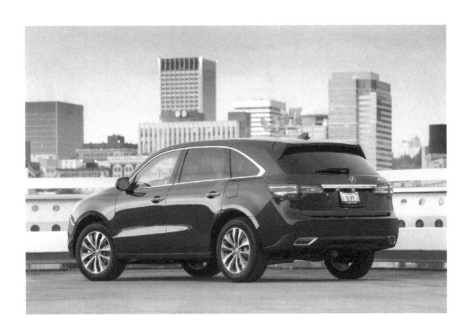

ACURA MDX – MDX is all-new for 2014. It seats seven, as it's one of the few luxury midsize SUVs with three rows of seats, although the third row is child-sized. A 3.5-liter V6 engine with a six-speed automatic transmission is standard, as is standard front-wheel drive; all-wheel drive is optional.

The new MDX body structure strikes a good balance between ride and handling while providing a much quieter ride. The interior is well designed with premium materials and uses a center stack touch screen instead of the former sea of buttons. If you want three rows, MDX is a good choice.

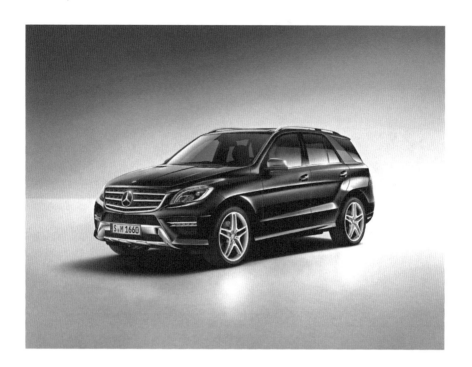

MERCEDES-BENZ M-CLASS – The SUV with the three-pointed star is sophisticated, solidly built, and enjoyable to drive. It offers a range of engine choices but the one that stands out is the diesel. The turbo diesel V6 in the ML350 BlueTEC is smooth, powerful, fuel-efficient, and worth paying for.

The M-Class has the most luxurious interior in the segment and while the AWD models will climb mountain trails or the highway, it's as comfortable as a limousine. Important safety options include a rear-view camera, active lane-keeping assist and park assist. Choose the classy comfort of the M-Class, as long as you don't need a third row.

LUXURY FULL-SIZE CARS

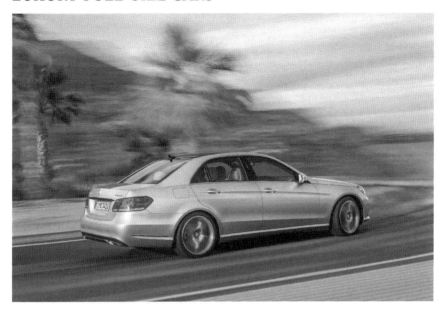

MERCEDES-BENZ E-CLASS – Handsome, comfortable, safe; it's no surprise that the E-Class leads the segment. The one you want is the Mercedes-Benz E250 BlueTEC, which comes with a turbo diesel, four-cylinder engine that has plenty of power for cruising, as well as acceleration for highway passing.

The E-Class' interior is most luxurious and combined with the solid ride, you feel like you're travelling in a well-upholstered bank vault. Safety is a given with Mercedes and standard on the E-Class is forward-collision warning and an Attention Assist system. Optional features include a rear-view camera, blind-spot monitoring, lane-departure warning, and adaptive cruise control.

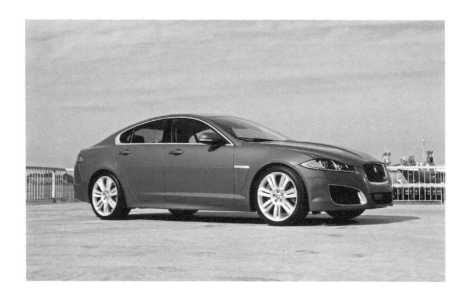

JAGUAR XF – The XF is the unique British alternative to more mainstream German and Japanese mid-size luxury sedans. It stands out for its stylishness, inside and out. It is a large sedan but it drives with the nimbleness of a smaller car through its extensive use of aluminum.

The 2014 Jaguar XF comes with a turbocharged four-cylinder engine, or a supercharged V6, or a supercharged V8. An eight-speed automatic transmission is standard in all models. The interior is magnificent and to emphasize its uniqueness – the shift knob rises out of the center console when you start the car.

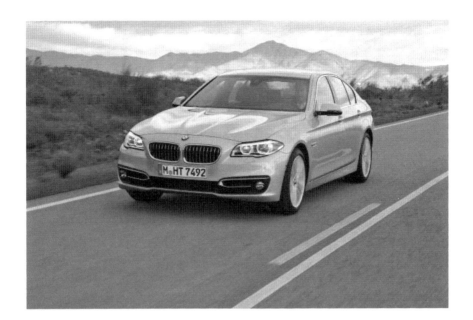

BMW 5 SERIES – The 5 Series now comes in sedan and hatchback body styles, five trim levels and five or six power train choices – rather bewildering. The base model has a turbocharged 2.0-liter four-cylinder engine and an eight-speed automatic transmission. Rear-wheel drive is standard, and all-wheel drive is optional.

It is now more of a luxury car than a performance car but it still has great driving dynamics for a car built for comfort. That comfort includes an elegantly plain but beautiful interior and perfect seats. The iDrive infotainment system is now finally easy to use. Forward-collision warning and blind-spot monitoring systems are optional.

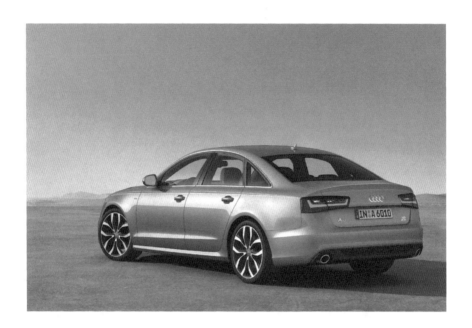

AUDI A6 – The A6 line-up begins with a turbocharged 2.0-liter four-cylinder engine, a continuously variable transmission (CVT), and front-wheel drive. But there are seven A6 versions in total, ranging up to a twin-turbocharged 4.0-liter V8 engine and all-wheel drive.

Audi A6 is known for two things; the best interiors in the class, with first-rate materials and a beautiful design, and a great driving experience. There are plenty of standard features while a rear-view camera, front and rear parking sensors, adaptive cruise control and a blind-spot monitoring system are options.

CHAPTER 8

Road Trips to Remember

The best way to travel for pleasure is by car. Maybe you have to take a plane to get to the car but once you're driving, you are free.

Now it's your schedule and your route. Go where you please and stop where you want. You've broken the chains of packaged holidays.

I'm going to outline fifteen of my favourite road trips from the last few years and stick to the ones that pack a great travel experience into a just a few days.

They all start, or can start, at a major airport. Take a Saturday layover at a major airport on your next vacation or business trip and you can save enough on airfare to cover the road trip.

Of the twelve, seven are in Europe. Driving in Europe is wonderful and easy to do. Car rentals, especially for smaller cars, are very reasonably priced. In England, of course, you're driving on the "wrong" side of the road but you get used to it quickly; just remember to concentrate every time you get on the road – that seems to be when mistakes are made.

Four great trips are in the U.S. and four are in Canada. In both countries, airport car rentals are an unbelievable bargain. Book ahead on the Internet, of course.

So, don't sit there – take a road trip. Feel the freedom of the open road.

If you take just one of these great trips, then the book has been worth it.

Heathrow to Windsor

Heathrow! The thought of London's main airport, the busiest one in Europe, triggers images of crowds, confusion, and delays. Ease your pain by taking a short overnight or even a day trip to nearby Windsor; the home of British royalty for the past nine centuries. It's amazing how few of my friends who are Heathrow regulars have ever travelled the mere twelve miles from the airport to Windsor.

If you have the rental car, follow the signs from Heathrow to the M4, head west (Reading and Bristol) and watch for the signs. Local bus service is also available from the airport.

The main attraction, of course, is Windsor Castle. It stands on a hill near the River Thames. A bridge over the Thames connects the town with Eton College; the school of the British establishment, founded in 1440. Eighteen Old Etonians have been Prime Minister.

The royals have been partial to Windsor since the first ones arrived in about 1086, probably in the reign of King Henry I. Things really got going about 300 years later; the construction of the castle under Edward III was the largest secular building project in England in the Middle Ages. As an early example of British supply-side economics, royal spending trickled down sufficiently to make the town one of the wealthiest in England.

Windsor hit a bit of a slump in the early 19th century, with the building of two army barracks. There was a major prostitution problem by 1830 and the town itself had been little improved since 1500. Things picked up in 1840 when Queen Victoria moved in. There was a big redevelopment of the castle (more trickle down) and two railways arrived. Windsor was transformed from a medieval has-been to the centre of the Empire.

Windsor Castle is the oldest and largest occupied castle in the world and one of the queen's official residences. She's usually there from April to June, plus the odd weekend. The State Apartments, the heart of the palace, are used for ceremonial and official occasions. They are furnished with some of the finest works of art from the Royal Collection, including paintings by Rembrandt, Rubens, and Van Dyck. In 1992, a fire raged for fifteen hours, destroying or damaging more than 100 rooms. Restoration work was completed in 1997 at a cost of more than $60 million.

Within the castle is St. George's Chapel, one of the finest examples of gothic architecture in England. The chapel is dedicated to the patron saint of the Order of the Garter, Britain's highest Order of Chivalry. It has been the setting for many royal weddings but not the one in 2005, between Prince Charles and the former Mrs. Parker Bowles. That took place across the street at Windsor's Guildhall. However, they dropped in to St. George's afterwards for an official blessing by the Archbishop of Canterbury, which was attended by about 800 family, friends and minor celebrities.

Tours of the castle are available daily for fifteen quid and well worth the time and cost. The scope of the tour depends on whether royals are on the premises or not. Check the top of the Round Tower. When the queen's there you'll see the Royal Standard flying; otherwise it's the Union Jack.

Windsor is linked to the town of Eton by pedestrian-only Windsor Bridge over the Thames. Eton College is the private school of choice for Britain's upper class. Approximately 1,300 boys-only, between the ages of 13 and 18 are boarders there. About 15% are from overseas; if you can get your kid in, tuition, room and board will cost about $50,000 for the year. The last Prime Minister from Eton, Sir Alec Douglas-Home, left office in 1964. Probably the most famous of all the Etonians was the Duke of Wellington, victor of Waterloo and later also Prime Minister.

Walking about the town and the college is a delightful way to spend an afternoon. History buffs will make discoveries at every turn. An example; architect Sir Christopher Wren, whose most famous work is St Paul's Cathedral in London, was a Windsor resident. He was asked to add pillars to the entrance to the Guildhall (the aforementioned wedding hall). Wren calculated that pillars were not necessary. He added the pillars as he was told, but to make his point, he left a gap at the top, so that the pillars do not actually support the roof. The building is still standing – a mere twelve miles from Heathrow airport agony.

Heathrow to The Peaks

Here's a slightly more ambitious road trip, to escape the horrors of Heathrow. It's a three-hour drive of about 170 miles, mostly up the M1. You're on your way to The Peaks.

The Peak District was established in 1951 as Britain's first national park. Fashionable it is not. This is the place where seedy Labourites in anoraks go hiking, while worrying about how to sustain the population of the water vole (a rat with a hairy tail). I'm not saying the water vole doesn't have a right to exist, I'm just trying to give you a flavour of the place. It's the kind of community that appeals to Prince Charles; he recently flew up in a helicopter (now that created some CO_2) to see how a local moorland restoration project is helping to combat global warming.

Although the Peak District is one of Britain's best-loved landscapes, there are actually no peaks – only hills, which are often covered with sheep. It is England's highland country at the south end of the Pennines. For hikers (no carbon footprint; be careful not to step on the water vole) this is perfection; from moorland, to grassy hills, to craggy rocks – all connected by public footpaths. Cars are not welcome.

This is where the "right to roam" was tested before it became law in Britain. In the 1930s, crowds of hikers walked defiantly across open land that belonged to the Dukes of Devonshire (more about them later). The leaders were arrested and imprisoned. In the 1950s, attitudes changed considerably, the National Park was created and the 11th Duke actually apologized to the "trespassers." Today, visitors can stroll almost anywhere, including the Duke's former estate of Chatsworth House. The pathways are ancient rights of way but the land over which they pass is invariably privately owned, so stay on the path or technically it's trespassing.

A National Park in Britain means that there are planning restrictions to protect the area from development but it doesn't mean that the land is owned by the government. As a result, there are plenty of attractive villages. The air is clear and bright as the terrain begins about a thousand feet above sea level.

The largest town is Buxton, developed in the eighteenth century by the Dukes of Devonshire, as a genteel health spa. The spa water, bubbling up from underground at a constant 83°F (28°C) has attracted health seekers since Roman times.

The town has a thriving arts scene and many fine buildings, including an elegant Edwardian Opera House that has something playing almost every night of the year. Buxton also features one of the oddest and most impressive buildings in England.

There's a huge dome (bigger than St Paul's in London) that was the largest unsupported dome in the world when built in 1785 as a stable for 110 horses. It was part of the reigning Duke's plan to promote Buxton as a spa. It remained a stable until 1881 when it was converted to a hospital. In 2001, it became part of the University of Derby, but the unmistakably spectacular dome remains intact.

Speaking of the Dukes of Devonshire, their historic home, Chatsworth House, is known locally as the Palace of the Peaks. It is the greatest of the District's stately homes and one of the greatest expressions of private wealth since the Elizabethan age. It has been the home of the Cavendish family (later titled) for more than 450 years.

They were able to keep up the place until the early 1950s when the 10th Duke died at the age of 55. At that point, death duties at the maximum rate of 80% had to be paid. Important works of art, as well as thousands of acres of land were sold. It still wasn't enough and in 1967, the ownership of the remaining estate passed to the Trustees of the Chatsworth Settlement in lieu of cash.

The family was allowed to move back in to the ground and first floors, for which the Duke pays rent. To cover the rest of the costs the house, the garden and the park is open for tours and special events. The district is famous for walks; there is no better one than on the grounds here.

If you're looking for a perfect escape to English countryside, away from the traffic jams of the south, point your airport rent-a-car to The Peaks.

Frankfurt to Vineyards of the Mosel

Frankfurt Airport, known locally as Flughafen Frankfurt am Main, is the largest airport in Germany and third largest in Europe. If you travel on Lufthansa, you're bound to have a stopover here.

Frankfurt is the financial center of Germany and as boring as only a financial centre can be. But airport rental cars are available and the no-speed-limit autobahn will get you out of town at an unbelievable velocity. It's a short dash to tour what I think is the most beautiful river in Europe and sample some Riesling wine from grapes grown in vineyards established by the Romans.

Follow the autobahn signs from the airport to Koblenz, about an hour at Mach 1. You'll cross the Rhine at that point but keep going in the direction of Luxembourg. Set your Navi, or buy a detailed road map of the Mosel - Eifel region at any gas station; you'll need one or the other. You're heading to the town of Cochem on the Mosel.

The Mosel (or Moselle in English or French) is a river in France and Luxembourg, which flows into Germany and joins the Rhine at Koblenz. It's 545 kilometers long but we're picking it up at about the halfway point.

Cochem's famous landmark is the 1,000-year-old castle. It was originally built in the 11th century but was completely destroyed by French soldiers in 1869. The present castle was rebuilt later in the 19th century; it towers above the river, which is known around the world for its brilliant scenery and fantastic wine.

The roads along the bank of the Mosel are ideal and separate bike paths run parallel. Perfect villages and vineyards greet you at every turn of this steep-sloped, meandering river. The Mosel carves its way through red slate, upon which are castles, abbeys, Roman sites, and stately homes. Vineyards and family-run gasthofs (small hotels) are everywhere along this unspoiled riverbank. Drive in the direction of Trier.

Trier is the oldest city in Germany, founded by the Roman Emperor Augustus in 15 BC. It has more important Roman remains than any other place in Northern Europe. Trier's Porta Nigra is the best-preserved Roman city gate north of the Alps and the huge Constantine Basilica was built as the throne hall of Roman Emperor Constantine. I spent hours in it, reading the excellent illustrated history that connects this building with two thousand years of German history.

Trier is certainly worth exploring but I don't recommend staying in this city of about 100,000 residents. Go back to the villages along the river. One nearby is Longuich, the site of a Roman villa, which is still partially standing.

Local knowledge is everything and I came to Longuich equipped with an introduction to a friend's family who have grown grapes and made sensational Riesling in this village for 203 years. The vineyards of the Carl Schmitt-Wagner Winery were purchased by the family in 1804 from the administration of Napoleon Bonaparte. They had previously belonged to a Benedictine Convent but has been secularized and then sold by the French invader. The Schmitt-Wagners knew that the clergy owned only the very finest vineyards so they paid Napoleon a hefty price. Since then, the Schmitt-Wagners have continued the old fashioned practices that have won their wine several important international awards.

The steep vineyards bordering the river have a sixty-degree pitch. They seemed vertical and I could barely stand there without sliding down the cliff. The Wagner-Schmitt family still tends nearly 6,000 ungrafted European vines that were planted by the family in 1896.

I spent the night in a village gasthof for the princely sum of 30 Euros (Cdn$43). The room was small and comfortable and as spotlessly clean and well prepared as any Four Seasons. In the morning, I launched the rental car back on the autobahn and made a warp-speed return to Frankfurt Flughaven. Songs are written about romance on the Seine or castles on the Rhine. I prefer a chilled glass of Riesling on the Mosel.

Munich to Mad King Ludwig's Castle

Munich is all about beer gardens, business, and BMW and after a day or two of that you'll need an escape. So, rent a car for a pleasant hour-long drive to an incredible, island palace on a beautiful alpine lake. It's part of the tale of Mad King Ludwig II of Bavaria.

In 1864 at the age of 18, Ludwig ascended, as they say, to the Bavarian throne. Not the least interested in democracy or modernism, Ludwig saw himself as the second coming of Louis XIV, the French Sun King, and decided he needed a palace the equal of Versailles. He drained Bavaria's Treasury to build it.

He selected an island in the middle of the Chiemsee, (pronounced keem-zay) Bavaria's largest lake. In 1878, after 10 years of planning, the construction of Herrenchiemsee began.

It was never completely finished but what was built is an amazing copy of the French original, lacking only the wings that make Versailles so immense. Ludwig's Hall of Mirrors actually exceeds the original in Versailles in size and grandeur. 2,000 candles, on elaborate chandeliers and candelabras, provide light.

You can visit Herrenchiemsee only on a guided tour. You enter through the monumental staircase inspired by the Duke's Palace in Venice. You pass through Ludwig's dining room that had a table hoisted, fully set, from the floor below so he could eat without servants bothering him. His bedchamber is a knock-off of the one the Sun King used for public ceremonies.

Throughout the palace, no surface was left ungilded or unadorned. The rooms are exact copies of their counterparts in Versailles, including paintings and sculptures. This is architectural plagiarism of the highest order and although only 20 of the planned 80 rooms were completed, it bankrupted the king.

The power brokers back in Munich weren't too pleased with the latest member of the Wittelsbach dynasty, which had ruled Bavaria for nearly eight centuries, and as construction continued for the tenth year, they had him declared him unfit to rule and removed him from the throne. Poor Ludwig drowned later that year, 1886, in suspicious circumstances. He had only spent a week living in his monument to Absolute Monarchy.

But Ludwig had been a busy boy during his brief reign. As well as Herrenchiemsee, he built beautiful castles at Neuschwanstein and Linderhof. And don't think architectural plagiarism died with Ludwig. You have likely seen Neuschwanstein before. It was ripped off by Disney's Magic Kingdom in Florida.

The ferry that takes you to the palace also stops on the neighbouring island of Fraueninsel, which has a Benedictine convent from the eighth century. It's a great spot for walks among the island's gardens and homes. Dine in an outdoor restaurant and admire the view of the Alps on the horizon.

Munich Airport is Europe's best and the connecting hub for many overseas flights. If you have a stopover, rent a car (make it a BMW because this is its home town) and take a pleasant 80-kilometer trip to Mad King Ludwig's Bavarian Versailles.

Rome to Pienza, Tuscany

If there is ever an airport from which you should escape, it is this one – Rome's Fiumicino, officially called Leonardo da Vinci Airport.

According to the Association of European Airlines, Fiumicino is the third worst airport in Europe, in terms of on-time performance (only Heathrow and Gatwick are worse, no surprise). But in terms of chaos, inefficiency, and rudeness, Fiumicino is my number one. So fight your way through the unruly mobs directly to the car rental counter and escape to a perfect Tuscan, Renaissance village. It's a fast 180 km trip, mostly on the northbound A1 Autostrada to the Valdichiana exit.

You're headed to Pienza, a hilltop village fit for a pope; in fact, it was created by a pope. Aeneas Piccolomini rose from obscurity to become Pope Pius II in 1458. He transformed his remote home village of Corsignano, south of Siena, into a Utopian Renaissance town, renaming it Pienza ("Pius-ville") in honour of himself.

By the way, if you've ever seen Franco Zeffirelli's 1968 film, *Romeo and Juliet*, you've seen Pienza, because it was mostly filmed on location there.

Pienza's in the centre of the Val d'Orcia, a beautiful, untouched valley. In 1996, UNESCO declared the town a World Heritage Site and in 2004 the entire valley was included on the list of UNESCO's World Cultural Landscapes. It is a scene of golden wheat, lavender, cypress trees, and stone farmhouses.

But getting back to Pope Pius II, he commissioned architect Bernardo Rossellino to build a Duomo (cathedral church) a papal palace, and a town hall. Construction started in about 1459. The main components were finished in only five years, followed by the rebuilding of the rest of the town.

The Duomo dominates the center of the piazza. It has had a fortune spent on it recently and is now in pretty good shape. Pius II wanted it to be a "a house of glass" to symbolize enlightenment in the Humanist age. It bears the scars from Second World War shelling. The palazzo is next door to the Duomo and was the home of Pius II's descendants until 1968. It is now open to the public and it provides spectacular views across to the wooded slopes of the Monte Amiata, the highest in Tuscany. Across from the church is the town hall, or Palazzo Comunale.

The village has a population of about 2,000 and is vehicle-free. It has one central street and numerous colourful alleys. You can also walk along the village's southern wall to take in the Val d'Orcia far down below. We had lunch in a little cafe on the wall itself.

Pienza's best hotel is Relais Chiostro di Pienza, which was a convent in the fifteenth century. It too overlooks the valley and has a very comfortable and well-stocked reading room on the main floor. Rooms run from about 100 to 200 Euros a night. Your other choice would be to stay at one of the many Agriturismo offerings, which are farmhouse and villa accommodations. We stayed at several in various parts of Italy and they were all more than satisfactory and surprisingly cheap.

There are numerous outdoor restaurants, cheese shops, artists' studios, and strategically located benches. Wherever there is a vista that you want to sit down and enjoy, you will find a bench located precisely on the spot to provide the most inspiring view.

You could spend weeks happily wandering around Tuscany, or ensconced in a villa, or just exploring Siena and Firenzi. But if you only have a day or two before facing the hell of Fiumicino, then Pienza's your best bet.

Barcelona to Sitges

Wisely you ask, "If I have a day or two to kill in Barcelona, why not stay there and enjoy what many tourist surveys consider the best city in Europe with its architecture, history, style, and nightlife?"

Um, well, er...you have a point. Barcelona has bounced back from a tortured history to become one of the liveliest cities on the Continent. Barcelona was a wasteland of ugly high-rises and industrial pollution during the years between the civil war and Franco's death. The Olympic Games were a catalyst for change as was a flood of EEC (European Economic Community) cash. Barcelona "turned itself around" to face the sea, creating a harbourfront and beach from former wasteland. And the museums and cathedrals (Gaudi's Sagrada Familia) and Las Ramblas have greater life than ever.

Wait a minute, I'm arguing against myself. There is a reason to leave Barcelona and get away from the traffic and commotion (it is a city of 1.5 million) and get closer to the Mediterranean. I discovered Sitges by riding a motorcycle about 40 km south down the C-246, a coastal road that clings precariously to the top of the seaside cliff.

Sitges is a popular resort and not nearly as tacky as Benidorm or Torremolinos. In fact, Sitges is called the St. Tropez of Spain, with property prices reflecting this status and the fact that it claims to have a unique microclimate with 300 sunny days a year. It has been a city of culture since the 19th Century, attracting the likes of Salvador Dalí and poet Federico García Lorca. The Spanish Civil War (1936-39) ended the "golden age" of Sitges.

Today it is also known as a summer party-town and in July and August the streets are crowded with affluent gays. I was there in spring and found the town utterly quiet and sedate.

The old part of Sitges is from medieval times and the castle is now the seat of the town government. The local parish church is built next to the sea at the town's highest point where an ancient stone stairway gives spectacular views. Narrow cobblestone streets lead to countless art galleries and two museums. Sitges has a population of about 30,000, of which a third come from other European countries.

The beaches are within the town. There is a long, wide sidewalk, which runs the length of the seafront. It's not exactly the Promenade des Anglais at Nice but it is lined with cafes and hotels, which face the blue Mediterranean. No shortage of good restaurants (all dishes seem to be combinations of fish and olives) and in late March there were plenty of empty tables. After dinner, around 11p.m., it was warm enough for a walk along the seafront sidewalk (Passeig Maritim), which is the palm-fringed corniche.

There are plenty of hotels; half of them in the four-star category. I stumbled upon one from the 19th-century, which is an old artists' hangout with every wall covered with paintings. There was outdoor dining under the palms and among the sculptures in the courtyard. I know, I know; Barcelona is so "in" right now, but don't miss Sitges.

Geneva to Rougemont, Switzerland

For spectacular Swiss skiing, my favourites are Wengen and Zermatt. But if you've finished your government agency meeting in Geneva (why else would you be there) and you want to find Alpine glory nearby, take a run to Rougemont.

You might not have heard of this town but you likely know of fashionable Gstaad just up the road. Rougemont is two hours (150km) from Geneva by car and two and a half hours by rail. In Switzerland, train travel is much more enjoyable.

Whether by car or by train, you'll travel the length of Lake Geneva to Montreux. Unless you're there in July, you'll miss the Jazz festival; but take a break there anyway. Montreux has beautiful walks along the lake and the town square features a statue of Freddie Mercury facing Lake Geneva. If you dig around a bit you can read about Queen and Deep Purple and Led Zeppelin and their history in Montreux. My recommendation is to take your time there and enjoy the lakeside walk, which is quite close to the train station.

When you re-join the train, you're on the Golden Pass railway line, part of the famous Montreux-Oberland-Bernois Railroad. This ancient line climbs vertically behind Montreux and cuts over the Alps. It departs from Montreux station on a slow switchback route, which leaves you hanging out over bottomless gorges. Once you get over the front range, you can enjoy the glass domes, panoramic cars that are perfect to take in the Swiss countryside. From Geneva the trip costs 73 Swiss francs, one way.

Rougemont (population less than 1,000) is located in the Pays d' Enhaut (high country) in the Canton of Vaud, up in the Alps. I have never seen a whole village of Swiss chalet architecture so well preserved.

The village is built along a single street, facing the valley and the sun. All the houses are of wooden construction, well over 100 years old, with gables, balconies, and decorative panels painted in bright colours. Its fabulous scenery and proximity to Geneva (and Gstaad) have driven real estate prices into the stratosphere. What I would consider a mid-market chalet was priced at 9 million Swiss Francs (that's approx. US$8million). The better chalets, higher up the mountain, are apparently occupied by Swiss pharma-billionaires. I am told that the great Duke Romanov, heir of the Russian tsar, also lives in exile in Rougemont.

The next village up the line (7 km west) is glamorous Gstaad, a fashionable jet-set destination surrounded by some of Switzerland's finest alpine scenery. In terms of skiing, it's no Zermatt, but it is an interesting area covering a vast terrain, which you can reach conveniently on the aforementioned Oberland-Bernois Railroad, which is included in your lift ticket.

The other way out of Rougemont, particularly on skis, is to take the Videmanette cable-car that runs from the village up to the high-country at 2186m. From there you can ski down to Gstaad. In fact there are more than 250 km of pistes in the area; get tired of one area and catch the train to the next.

Don't be put off by Gstaad's glittering, ultra-expensive reputation. It is a pleasant, car-free, one-street village, which happens to be packed with the jewellers' shops and furriers that attract Europe's royal households and various hangers-on. While Gstaad is Five Star expensive (a weathered wooden chalet there costs more than $10,000,000 according to recent listings) Rougemont has more charm.

Rougemont might be relatively down-market but it does have direct access to the mountains and a great little ski shop for rentals so you don't have to drag your skis around. There are three small hotels in town, friendly places with excellent Swiss cooking. Expect about $250 a night for two with breakfast. After a day on the slopes and a chalet evening you can easily make it back to Geneva airport by road or rail for a midday flight home.

Back Door to Palm Springs

Thousands travel the 105 miles (nobody knows what a kilometre is out here) from LA to Palm Springs each week, to enjoy desert sunshine in the old hang-out of Frank Sinatra, Bob Hope, and boozy movie stars of the past. The normal trip is straight out I-10, driving as fast as you can, turn right into the town. But there is a much, much better route for a driver.

You start out on I-10 but only until you get to Banning, California (80 miles) and then turn right on Route 243. Ahead of you is a 66-mile, two-lane highway that climbs from Banning over the scenic San Jacinto Mountains and eventually down to the outskirts of Palm Springs in the Coachella Valley.

Route 243 is known as the Banning-Idyllwild Panoramic Highway and it's a 30-mile drive from Banning to Idyllwild. A little farther on, it meets Route 74, which is known as The Palms to Pines Highway (you will indeed be traveling Pines to Palms). Put the two together and you have the very best drive in California, even better than the famous US-1 along the Pacific coast, according to *AutoWeek* Magazine.

So, let's start at Banning where you turn off I-10 and starting climbing and climbing. Elevations rise from 2,400 feet above sea level at Banning to 6,165 feet at Pine Cove and 5,400 at Idyllwild. It is a winding mountain road with great vistas at every turn and lots of places to pull off and go for a walk. Most of the route lies within the San Bernardino National Forest and this section of road is known locally as the "Esperanza Firefighters Memorial Highway," in memory of five firefighters who died fighting a huge wildfire here in 2006.

The only real town along the way is Idyllwild, a very artsy place with backwoods hippies and painters and potters in equal numbers. It's on a ridge in the San Jacinto Mountains among tall pines and cedars and has certainly kept its small town atmosphere with locally owned shops and restaurants. In the centre of town is the Idyllwild Tree Monument, a 50-foot totem pole. The winter population is about 3,000 but it more than doubles in the summer as the heat sends city people to the higher elevations of their vacation homes. Idyllwild is also well known with the rock climbing crowd. The Suicide Rocks are particularly popular, for reasons that escape me completely.

Up to this point, you've been passing through forested mountainsides with pine, oak, and fir and a number of protected areas of wildlife habitat. You've had sweeping views with snow-capped mountains in the distance. All the California ad agencies shoot car commercials on this road and Elvis Presley even shot a movie up here called *Kid Galahad* – I never saw it.

But past Idyllwild, you begin to descend to the desert. First, you travel through the ranch country of the foothills and then into arid brush and cactus-covered desert. You will have descended about 1200 feet by the time you reach the town of Pinyon Pines and then you really start to drop. You have to lose nearly four thousand feet vertical before you reach Palm Springs. You have lots of switchback turns to negotiate while being distracted by the fabulous views of the desert below.

You get back to "civilization" as you enter Palm Desert, really a Palm Springs suburb and one of those places that grew like crazy before the housing bubble burst. Thousands of aging baby-boomers have places here, including Bill Gates. Press on through the six-lane roads that could be Anywhere, USA until you reach Palm Springs. Pull up to the Gene Autry Hotel (now called Le Parker), lounge by the pool, order a pitcher of martinis and pretend it's 1963.

Denver to the Ski Slopes

In Canada, we're all crazy about skiing at Whistler because the Olympics were there – but it does rain a lot. That's why you should never sell Colorado short as a ski destination.

Colorado is the home of the 14-ers. The state has 54 peaks that rise higher than 14,000 feet, while all of Canada has only 15 such mountains. Colorado has another 1,140 peaks, which are over 10,000 feet – so you're getting the picture and it's a good one for skiers.

This road trip begins at Denver International Airport, which gets my vote for the best airport in North America. It should be good; it opened in 1995, 16 months behind schedule and nearly $2 billion over budget. It occupies twice as much land as all of Manhattan. Make your way to the car rental counters in the gateway terminal; that's the one with a distinctive white fabric roof designed to look like the snow-capped Rockies just down the road.

The hard-core skier might insist on Telluride, but it's 330 miles away. There's fantastic skiing within an easy drive of the airport gates and let's start with Breckenridge (98 miles away), which features four massive peaks.

Breck bills itself as the highest resort in America. On my first morning there, in bright sunshine and tons of snow, I found myself a little short of breath. Then I noticed I was skiing at an elevation of 11,059 feet (3,372m) on Peak 8. In a small aircraft, you're required to have bottled oxygen once you get up to 10,000 feet. In Breck's back bowls you may want that oxygen when you find runs with confidence-inspiring names like "Psychopath" and "Bone Yard" and double diamond blacks galore.

The town of Breckenridge sells itself as a 150-year-old, quaint Victorian town. The old part is pleasant enough but the rest of it is a condo, time-share monolith. I have a better idea about where to stay.

But let's continue with our drive-to-skiing first with a visit to Vail, the largest ski area in North America. This one stretches 7 miles end to end and is one of the Grand Dames of western skiing since it was founded in 1962. Don't worry, it has been constantly upgraded and improved since then. The lift system is ultra-modern and goes everywhere. Lots of sunshine and no lift lines; you can't ski this place out in a day. In 1972, Vail and nearby Beaver Creek were slated to host the ski events of the 1976 Winter Olympic Games. However, the voters of Colorado shot down the idea and the Winter Games went to Innsbruck, Austria instead.

Vail's marketing message today is that it brings Alpine charm to the American Rockies. Zermatt it isn't. To me, Vail looks more like a massive concrete resort plunked down beside the highway (I-75) and dressed up in Swiss clothes. But the skiing is definitely of Alpine quality.

One more ski stop, then lodging. Arapahoe Basin should not make the list for novice skiers in Colorado. This place has been around since 1946, when a rope-tow was installed mid-mountain and a military truck hauled skiers up to it.

Now it has more than 100 trails and multiple chairlifts, with high alpine, groomed runs, bowls, chutes, and glades. The skiing is challenging and the lift tickets are cheap, but off the slopes Arapahoe is pretty miserable. The "village" at the foot of the slopes is a glorified shelter with a lunch counter and ski shop. But it gives you a taste of the early days of this sport.

Now that I've panned Breck and Vail villages, where can you stay? Try the mountain town of Frisco, just down the road from Breckenridge. Frisco is a mining town from the 1880s that is remarkably intact and original. This is not Five Star Deluxe Vail by any means, but a thoroughly pleasant little town in a beautiful mountain setting. There are several inns and restaurants to keep you going for another day on the slopes or that easy ninety-minute drive back to Denver International.

The Road to Boston

Canadians with a sense of history, who don't mind being referred to as "tyrants" and "oppressors" (by Americans yet), might travel to Boston, Massachusetts.

The Birthplace of the American Revolution has historic site upon site, celebrating the defeat of hated British colonizers and sympathizers, many of whom were expelled northward to Canada. It's interesting and inflammatory reading but fortunately, the Red Sox / Blue Jays wars are taken more seriously by Bostonians these days.

Boston is perfect for a short summer vacation and as with any good road trip, the "drive" is the best part. Start your drive to Boston in the direction of Gananoque, not toward Niagara Falls or Fort Erie. You're heading for the Thousand Islands Bridge System (four bridges, four islands), which extends from Ivy Lea near Gananoque, Ontario to the US side near Alexandria Bay, NY, providing a direct connection between Highway 401 and US Interstate Rt. 81.

The view of the woods and waters from my Mini Cooper S convertible was spectacular. Enjoy the crossing because your first side trip is just ahead. Once off the last bridge, watch for signs to Clayton, NY, which is the home of the Antique Boat Museum, North America's largest collection of freshwater recreation boats. There are more than 100 examples of the fabulous mahogany launches and race boats owned by the millionaires, who once summered in great style along the St. Lawrence River. It's the best museum of its kind in the world.

From Clayton you can pick up the signs for Sackets Harbour.

Sheltered on Black River Bay, the historic village of Sackets Harbour was the headquarters for the US Navy on the Great Lakes during the War of 1812 with Great Britain, which is known as the "Second War of Independence." During that war, one-third of the United States Army and a quarter of its Navy was stationed at Sackets Harbour. Today, the village is one of New York State's Heritage Areas with exceptional historic attractions and beautiful tree-lined streets. If staying over, the Ontario Place Hotel is acceptable.

Head back to Rt. 81 and travel southward to Syracuse. Then it's time to take your toll ticket and get on the New York State Thruway. It joins directly onto the Mass Turnpike and you'll be paying toll every inch of the way from here to the Massachusetts border (270 miles; US$10.95) if you don't get off. But you will get off, just not for a while. Take the New York State Thruway (I-90) to Exit 30 Herkimer (57 miles; $2.25) then take Route 28 South for 30 miles to Cooperstown.

On the way, you will pass Glimmerglass Opera's Alice Busch Opera Theater, built on 43 acres of donated farmland, which opened in June 1987. The 900-seat theater is notable for its beautiful setting on the shore of Otsego Lake. Sliding walls allow the audience to enjoy fresh air and views of the surrounding countryside before performances and during intermissions. Glimmerglass has grown to international stature and now offers 43 performances of four operas each season.

But this trip's for baseball, not baritones, and ten minutes farther down the road is the National Baseball Hall of Fame. This is a superb sports museum and a baseball fan can spend hours and hours in the exhibitions and permanent collections. It's open every night until 9:00p.m. and the evening is the best time to visit after the crowds have returned to the trailer parks. Yes, there are those around Cooperstown and the main street has a bit of a baseball carnival atmosphere. But overall it is a very pleasant town on the southern end of Otsego Lake, the "Glimmerglass" of James Fenimore Cooper's *Leatherstocking Tales*.

Back out to the New York Thruway now, to continue east through the Mohawk Valley and along the Mohawk River. This is the natural route, which connected traders on the Atlantic seaboard with the continental interior. The valley was the scene of important Revolutionary War battles and ongoing skirmishes between Loyalists and Patriots. The Erie Canal, completed in 1825, loosely follows the course of the Mohawk River. For thruway driving it's most enjoyable.

Shortly after crossing the mighty Hudson River east of Albany, you'll reach the Massachusetts border and enter the Berkshire Hills. Take the second exit for Lee and Lenox, Massachusetts to find the Tanglewood Music Center, the summer home of the Boston Symphony Orchestra and the setting for a wide variety of musical performances. The bluebloods of Boston come here with their gourmet picnic baskets and listen to live music as the sun sets and the stars twinkle.

Back to the Mass Pike for the final 130 miles into Boston. Boston is one of America's oldest cities, first incorporated in 1630. Boston likes to think of itself as a center for social and political change. The city itself has about 590,000 residents and in the Greater Boston area are several institutions of higher education, including Harvard and M.I.T.

Boston is a great city for walking and the Freedom Trail is a perfect introduction to Colonial Revolutionary Boston. The trail takes you to 16 historical sites at your own pace; a red brick or painted line connects the sites on the trail and serves as a guide.

The starting point is the Boston Common, one of the oldest public parks in the country. Cattle grazed the common and until 1817, public hangings took place here. British troops camped on Boston Common prior to the Revolution.

Farther along the trail, in front of the Old State House, a circle of cobblestones commemorates the Boston Massacre of March 5, 1770. British soldiers faced an angry crowd of colonists, who hurled snowballs, rocks, clubs, and insults. The soldiers fired into the crowd and killed five colonists. Samuel Adams and other patriots called the event a "massacre." Loyal "tyrants" and "oppressors" beware.

Two Boston neighbourhoods well worth exploring are the unimaginatively named North End and South End. The North End is most famous for its Italian restaurants and strong Italian roots. The church that hung the lanterns to signal Paul Revere can be found here. The South End has blocks and blocks of original Victorian brick rowhouses, upscale restaurants, and art galleries. It reminds me of that section of downtown Saint John, New Brunswick, which remains intact but the South End is much bigger and glitzier.

Car enthusiasts will want to check out The Larz Anderson Auto Museum, located in Larz Anderson Park in nearby Brookline. A magnificent carriage house, built in the 1880s to resemble a French chateau, has been transformed into a showcase for the beautiful automobiles that Larz Anderson began collecting in Paris in 1899. During the next 50 years, he purchased at least thirty-two new motorcars, in addition to numerous carriages, creating America's oldest motorcar collection.

You can view automobiles made by; Delahaye, Delage, Facel-Vega, Voisin, Renault, Citroen, DeDion, Leon Bollee, Bugatti, Peugeot, Rochet-Schneider, Gardner-Serpollet and many more.

Drive down again sometime and I'll tell you about the Boston Harbour Islands and the sailing at Marblehead and how I got a ticket for Fenway Park. One good road trip deserves another.

The Henry Ford

A few years ago, I had just finished a 10-hour day of interviews at Ford world headquarters in Dearborn, Michigan. The PR people wanted us to make a side trip up the road to "The Henry Ford," for a ride in a Model T. It was, after all, the 100th anniversary of the car that put America on the road.

"Oh no," I whined. "Another American theme park; let's skip it." But our enthusiastic guide insisted that we press on and I'm glad we did.

The Henry Ford, also known as the Henry Ford Museum and Greenfield Village, is a National Historic Landmark that preserves the character of the American Industrial Revolution. There's everything there from Thomas Edison's laboratory, to the Wright Brothers' bicycle shop, to the limousine in which John F. Kennedy was shot.

The museum began as Henry Ford's personal collection of historic objects. Today it is a huge (49,000 m^2) display of antique machinery, cars, locomotives, aircraft, and pop culture icons.

Greenfield Village is next door and nearly a hundred historical buildings were moved there, to show how Americans have lived and worked since 1776. Its 240 acres (970,000 m^2) includes an operating steam railway and pasture for the sheep and horses.

The displays are brilliant and the informational content is thorough; there is no hucksterism or hype. I could easily spend a whole day there and I'm a very impatient traveler.

After nearly not enough time in the museum, we walked over to the village to take a spin in the car that made Henry famous. The Model T, built from 1908 until 1927, remains one of the top-selling vehicles of all time. More than 16 million were sold during its lifetime and nearly 12 million of them were black. Painting them one colour saved money on the assembly line, which enabled Henry to pay workers the unexpectedly large salary of five dollars a day.

If you go to this most un-Disney-like attraction, you will have the option of traveling around the place in a horse-drawn omnibus, a steam locomotive, a 1931 Model A, or one of the many Ford Model Ts.

There are a number of special events each summer, including a Ragtime Street Fair with jazz, parades, and food from the early 20th century. The Detroit Symphony Orchestra also performs patriotic music here at various times.

I hate theme parks and the idea of a roadside attraction causes a detour in the other direction. I was suspicious about the Henry, but it turned out to be a most worthwhile stop.

If you're interested, the Henry Ford is about 10 miles south of Detroit, via Interstates 75, 96 and 94, in that order. The address is 20900 Oakwood Blvd., Dearborn, MI; the website is thehenryford.org.

The Crowsnest Highway

In 1882, William Cornelius Van Horne decided that the Canadian Pacific Railway must take the shortest route across the Rockies and he chose the Rogers Pass. In 2006, you, on the other hand, should choose the Crowsnest Pass for your Rocky Mountain driving vacation.

Scheduled train service through the Rogers Pass started in June 1886. The TransCanada Highway also follows this original CPR route and road construction through the pass was completed in 1962. Rogers Pass (elevation 4,534 feet/1382 m) may be the TransCanada Highway's crowning glory, with five long tunnels to protect you from avalanches.

The Crowsnest Pass is farther south and it was completed in 1898, providing access to large areas of southern Alberta and south-eastern British Columbia. The Crowsnest Highway, designated as Highway

3, runs from the British Columbia-Alberta border in the Rockies, through the Crowsnest Pass and all the way west to Hope B.C. at the east end of the Fraser Valley (1,163 km; 722 miles).

The great majority of highway travelers bound for Vancouver, including nearly all the big transport trucks, simply head west from Calgary to Banff and on through the Rogers Pass. If you're planning the western tour this summer, I'd recommend the southern route.

Drive south from Calgary to join Highway 22, sometimes called the Cowboy Trail. You'll pass through the sister towns of Turner Valley and Black Diamond, which were once important oil and gas centres but now are home to cattle-ranching financiers from Calgary. The drive becomes even more beautiful toward Longview (say hello to Ian Tyson if you see him) on the way to Pincher Creek near the Crowsnest Pass. Think of the Alberta Provincial flag with wheat fields, ascending to foothills, ascending to snow-capped peaks – you're driving it.

I'm not strenuously opposed to driving the TC (TransCanada Highway #1). But when you're out here in ranchland, with hardly a car in sight, you'll be happy you're not dodging the trucks and trailers and campers on the Calgary-Banff speedway.

On to Crowsnest Pass, an area developed as a major coal supply area for early twentieth-century railroad and steel industries. Highway 3 takes you past the site of one of the world's biggest rock slides, the Frank Slide of 1903 and Canada's worst mining disaster, Hillcrest in 1914. As you cross the British Columbia border, you're heading for Fernie.

An annual average of 8.8 metres (29 feet) of powder snow buries Fernie's five alpine bowls in the majestic limestone cliffs of the Lizard Range. This is one of the great ski resorts in Canada but it is not lacking in summer activities, ranging from the ubiquitous golf, to lots of local art. Plenty of accommodation here and you might want to make it your first night's stop.

The road to Cranbrook in the Purcell Mountains beckons. I recently drove this stretch early on a Sunday morning. The air was fresh, the scenery magnificent and the road, with its ascents and descents and sweeping curves, gave my little Honda Civic Si a terrific workout. What an amazing little car. If you were blindfolded (I'm not suggesting it), on the high-speed stretches in 5th and 6th gears, you'd swear you were in a BMW or even a Porsche. Nice work Honda.

Cranbrook is known for hockey players and the Canadian Rail Museum. The museum is a work in progress. You jog south now, almost to the US border to Creston where you make a decision. Make this decision. Take the road north (3A) along the east side of Kootenay Lake. This is the most beautiful body of water in Canada (not beside Canada but inside Canada). Great road – spectacular vistas – last of the hippies in charming hamlets. Then the free bonus! BC Ferries runs a series of inland ferries and the one across Kootenay Lake toward Nelson is the best free boat ride I can ever remember. Don't miss it. Or Nelson for that matter. Nelson is a beautifully preserved city that has prospered from BC's most famous yet illegal crop.

Continue on to Castelgar, Christina Lake, and Grand Forks. I barely saw a car past Castelgar and my rate of progress was in inverse proportion to the amount of traffic. Another northward loop around mountains into ranch country again. Mmmm, what are real estate prices like here? And get ready for the mighty descent into Osoyoos. Lots of hotels in this town if you need a stop.

Welcome to the Southern Okanagan – Canada's pocket desert. The sweep of the irrigation sprinklers has transformed it into magnificent orchards and vineyards. The sprinklers also seem to keep the rattlesnakes distracted.

A story now. In the late '70s, two engineers from the University of Waterloo headed west to spend the rest of their days in a miserable oil field somewhere. They suffered through the Trudeau-induced collapse of the industry, got some wind in their sales in the '90s and emerged (one of them in particular) stinking rich. What do rich people aspire toward these days? Vineyards and wineries of course. That's where several of the California dotcom billions went too.

The money in question here became Tinhorn Creek Estate Winery (www.tinhorn.com), which is on the "bench" a little north of Osoyoos near Oliver. Wow! Am I back in Margaret River in Western Australia? Or is this "premier cru" territory in Medoc? What beauty. Our engineers-made-good put me up in a little guesthouse they keep in the midst of the grapes with the South Okanagan's best view.

From Osoyoos you're blasting westward through the edges of the desert on your way to Princeton. Fabulous, lightly traveled roads climbing back onto higher ground with only the curves and the elevation changes to keep you from another land speed record. Princeton is the start of the Princeton-Hope highway, which takes you through Manning Provincial Park. There's a nice place to stay if you need an overnight.

You'll also enjoy the drive to Hope and on to Chilliwack. Follow the traffic. Look out for the Mounties. It'll give you a taste of what it's like going through Banff these days. Drive directly to the Sylvia Hotel (built in 1912) on Vancouver's English Bay. Book a room, have a cold beer in the bar with the view. Now walk across the street and dip your toes in Pacific waters. Van Horne had the right destination in mind. He was just a bit early to know which would be the better drive.

Manitoulin Island

Manitoulin means Spirit Island in the Ojibwa language. Here's a terrific thousand-kilometer road trip that will take you through Manitoulin's Rainbow Country while you enjoy driving some of the most scenic roads in Ontario.

As I'm sure you know, Manitoulin is the world's largest island in freshwater. It's located in Lake Huron north of the Bruce Peninsula; both the Bruce and Manitoulin are extensions of the Niagara Escarpment.

The Bruce Trail is the public footpath that spans the entire escarpment (850km Niagara Falls to Tobermory) and you will have time to get out of the car for a short hike on one of its most beautiful sections.

Begin by heading toward Owen Sound – take Highway 6 or 10, your choice, then north to Wiarton. Highway 6 continues up the middle of the Bruce Peninsula but turn off either toward the Lake Huron side or the Georgian Bay side. This time let's go toward the Bay on Road 9. Take your time; you have to catch the ferry in Tobermory but don't try to make it on Day One.

You are in a World Biosphere Reserve and near two National Parks – Bruce Peninsula and Five Fathom. Enjoy the massive cliffs with thousand-year-old cedar trees overhanging the clear waters of Georgian Bay. Look for hidden coves with a sandy beach. Stop in Lion's Head and Dyer's Bay, which are villages hugging the limestone cliffs. From Dyer's Bay you can hike to the Cabot Head Lighthouse. There is also a short 3km loop that takes you up to the edge of the escarpment with dramatic views of forest and bay.

Tobermory is the fishing village that is the home base of the ferry that runs to Manitoulin Island. Try the local meal of whitefish and chips. The ferry runs from Little Tub Harbour, which has boats and ferries and shops and restaurants. Big Tub Harbour is much quieter and has beautiful cottages and the Big Tub Lighthouse at the entrance.

You have reserved your space on the Chi-Cheemaun, which means "big canoe" in the Ojibwa language. It's the Ontario Northlands ferry that runs four times a day, carrying 113 vehicles and 638 passengers for the 2-hour, 50- kilometre journey across to the island. It costs roughly $30 per car and $12 per passenger and provides perfect views of Flowerpot Island and Cove Island on your way across the Channel.

Like the Bruce Peninsula, Manitoulin Island is limestone, with high rocks along its north side and flatlands sloping into Lake Huron to the south. It is about half the size of Prince Edward Island and contains more than 100 lakes. Manitoulin is 160 km long and its width varies from 3 to 64 km. The island was a sacred place for the native people and travelers today write about the spirituality they feel when they cross the waters.

The North Channel of Lake Huron is the northern shore of Manitoulin Island, which today is one of the finest sailing areas in the world and the northern gateway to the Thirty Thousand Islands. This was part of the route used by the voyageurs to reach Lake Superior.

Champlain met the Odawa people here in 1615. The Jesuits set up a mission near Wikwemikong, in 1648. Diseases introduced by Europeans had a devastating effect on the island's population. According to legends, the island was burned to purify it and remained largely unsettled for the next 150 years.

Native people began to return following the War of 1812. The island was ceded to the Crown in 1836; however the Wikwemikong chief did not accept this treaty and that reserve remains unceded. Wikwemikong Unceded Indian Reserve occupies the large peninsula on the eastern end of Manitoulin Island, accessible across the isthmus between Manitowaning Bay and South Bay.

The ferry lets you off in South Baymouth and you should drive toward Providence Bay. On the way, look for signs to Michael's Bay, which is a spectacular, undeveloped beach known to surfers across North America. Providence Bay has cabins and a sandy beach popular with children who don't mind cold water.

On Manitoulin, you will find small, family-run resorts and restaurants, plenty of local crafts and absolutely none of the big travel chains. If you want the traffic and the glamour and the prices of Muskoka, you have come to the wrong place.

To give you an idea of what to expect, nightlife here is the activity of the Manitoulin Island Dark Sky Association. Their mission is to preserve the beauty of the night sky for future generations by establishing Manitoulin Island as a "National Dark Sky Sanctuary."

Continue along Road 542 to Gore Bay, which is a perfect harbour between two tree-covered bluffs for the big yachts traveling to or from the North Channel. Continue on at your leisure to Kagawong and then to Little Current.

Little Current is Manitoulin's gateway community from Northern Ontario and your departure point. You will cross the town's most famous landmark; the swing bridge. It was built as a railway bridge in 1913. After the Second World War, it was modified for vehicles. The bridge swings open for about 15 minutes on the hour, in daylight during the summer, to let boats pass through the channel.

Turn north onto Highway 6 toward Espanola and the Trans-Canada Highway. You will twist and turn through the La Cloche Mountains of the Canadian Shield, some of them very white, with views of local lakes and towns. Pick up the TC (Highway 17), bypass Sudbury (on this trip), and head south on Highway 69. Find the turnoff for Highway 637, which runs about 60 kilometres to Killarney. You'll pass dozens of lakes and rivers and sharply rising hills that look like small mountains. You'll do double-takes on the ones that are capped with snow-white outcroppings of quartzite. The evergreens on the hills make the resemblance to snow all the stronger.

Killarney is one of the oldest villages in Northern Ontario. By the 1750s, this was a major water route for the French fur traders. Located at the entrance of the North Channel, Killarney is famous for cruising waters, sea kayaking routes, and the pink granite islands. Rent a boat and visit some.

Six kilometers from the village is Killarney Provincial Park, considered the crown jewel of Ontario's park system. George Lake at the main park entrance provides calm waters for canoeists and a sand beach for swimming.

After a night or two in Killarney, you're ready for the drive home. Circle completed, another great road trip in the book.

Rideau Waterway

Here's an easy road trip for a summer swim; or you can tuck it away for later and take in the fabulous fall colours. It's a relaxing journey along the Rideau Waterway – a series of lakes, rivers, canals and locks that connects the Ottawa River at Ottawa to Lake Ontario at Kingston.

The Rideau was built by the British between 1826 and 1831, under the direction of Lieutenant Colonel John By and the Royal Engineers, as part of the British defense of North America. The need for an inland supply route had been seen in the War of 1812 when the American navy attacked British supply ships traveling up the St. Lawrence River from Montreal to the Great Lakes. The waterway is 202 kilometres long, including 19 kilometres of canals. It was opened in May 1832, making it the oldest continuously-operated canal system in North America.

Of course things settled down between Canada and the United States and the Rideau was never used as a military supply route. There was even talk of dismantling it in the early 20th century.

Now the Rideau system is a designated Canadian Heritage River and a nominated World Heritage Site. Most of the locks are operated by hand, just as they were in 1832, and the whole system is run by Parks Canada.

There are many towns and villages nestled along the Rideau and we'll begin our tour just north of Kingston. Take the 401 exit at Kingston called Montreal Street and turn north; start watching immediately for signs pointing east to Kingston Mills.

At Kingston Mills, the Cataraqui River falls about 6 metres over a series of rocky falls (Cataraqui Falls). High cliffs line the river as it descends toward Lake Ontario at Kingston Bay. This is the first lock station in the southern part of the Rideau, and you'll see a flight of 3 locks, a turning basin, and an upper lock. There's a blockhouse, one of only four built along the Rideau, which has a commanding view of both the north and south approaches to the lock.

After hiking around this impressive site, go back to "Montreal Street" and continue north. You'll pass through Sunbury and Battersea on your way to Jones Falls. When you get there, be sure to take the walk into the engineering marvel that is Jones Falls Dam. It is a magnificent stone arch dam, 20-metres-high, which was the largest dam in North America when constructed 180 years ago.

The construction of the dam and locks at Jones Falls was one of the great challenges faced by the builders of the canal. They had to overcome a series of rapids more than a kilometre long. Four locks were necessary at the site, each with a lift of five metres.

You can overnight at Jones Falls, but don't expect the Four Seasons. The original hotel was built in 1849 and burned down; Thomas Kenney constructed the present Hotel Kenney in 1888. It's a classic turn-of-the-century resort with three floors of balconies with railings. In 1910, renovations added the third story and as far as I can tell, improvements stopped then. But don't be deterred; staying there is like stepping back in time.

From Jones Falls, continue on Road 11 (the one you arrived on) east to Highway 15 and then north. Up ahead at Road 9, turn off for Chaffey's Lock. You can visit Chaffey's Lock Master's House Museum and check out the Opinicon Hotel, which is one of Eastern Ontario's oldest resorts. It has been owned and operated by the same family since 1921 and retains its 19th Century grandeur.

Back to Highway 15 and north to the turn at Highway 42, which leads to Newboro and Westport. Newport occupies the isthmus between the Rideau and Newboro Lakes. Here a lock was constructed and a channel excavated that linked the waters of the Rideau River System flowing northward to Bytown (now Ottawa) and the Cataraqui System flowing southward toward Kingston. Cutting through the hard rock of Canadian Shield granite just beneath the surface proved to be one of the most difficult tasks undertaken on the canal. Many lives were lost to accidents and malaria.

Westport is located at the west end of Upper Rideau Lake and has craft shops and eclectic art galleries. From here, pick up Road 8 north and follow it to Perth.

After the War of 1812, Perth was established as part of that defense plan against invasion from the south. The streets of this scenic, one-square-mile village, set along the Tay River, are lined with heritage homes and shops. The Tay Canal was completed in 1887, to connect Perth to the main Rideau system.

From here you can head into Ottawa to see the Rideau Canal's northern entrance from the Ottawa River. The Ottawa Locks consists of a flight of eight locks, which sits right between the Parliament Buildings and Chateau Laurier Hotel.

But I think that's for a separate trip and I'd suggest you take Highway 1 from Perth to Rideau Ferry. In the 1890s, a number of summer homes were established here on the south shore of the Lower Rideau Lake. You can enjoy the beach at the Rideau Ferry Conservation Area. The former Rideau Ferry Yacht Club donated this 10-acre shoreline property in 1976. Then continue on to Lombardy where you meet Highway 15 again and head south.

The next town is Portland, which was established in the early 1820s. Then it was known as "the Landing" as it was the major stepping-off point for those intending to homestead in the Perth area. The completion of the Rideau Canal in 1832 turned Portland into a thriving village of trade and transhipment. It was pretty well over by 1900 as the railways advanced, but Portland remains today the centre of cottage life on Big Rideau Lake. You can rent everything from houseboats to cruisers to canoes and kayaks at Portland. And you'll probably find one available; the Rideau Canal system has been hard hit this season by high gas prices, bad weather and tie-ups at the US border. Marina owners say boat traffic is down by as much as 30% this year.

At this point, you can continue down Highway 15 to Kingston and the 401. Better still, take out the map and explore more of the winding roads of this historic area of Upper Canada.

Loyalist Parkway to the Thousand Islands

Here's an enjoyable round trip of about 700 km from Toronto, which will let you follow the footsteps of the United Empire Loyalists as you travel the shoreline of Lake Ontario to the famous Thousand Islands.

Make a fast start on the 401 to Exit 522 (Wooler Road), which is between Brighton and Trenton. Feel free to travel instead on Highway 2 through the towns of Port Hope and Cobourg. There are plenty of signs pointing to The Loyalist Parkway, which you will follow for about 90 km from this point to Kingston.

After the American Revolution of 1776, those who had supported Britain were persecuted and had their property, and often their lives, taken by Americans of the new republic. Survivors fled to areas of British protection in western Quebec and eastern Ontario. The settlers suffered but persevered to help form Ontario and ultimately Canada. The Loyalist Parkway is their memorial.

Quinte's Isle is Prince Edward County. You will be joining it across the only land link from the mainland (there are also two bridges) and you will be leaving it eventually on a ferry. The county borders the Bay of Quinte on the north and Lake Ontario on the south with about 800 km of ever-changing coastline in total. It has recently been discovered to be a promising wine-producing region and that has brought with it the forces of gentrification with vineyards, wineries, and thoroughbred horses; the "mink and manure" crowd is gaining a foothold. But you are here to enjoy the unspoiled countryside and great swimming. At Sandbanks Provincial Park on the shore of Lake Ontario you will explore the huge sand dunes and golden beaches of the largest freshwater sandbar in the world. There is no shortage of high quality inns and B&Bs in the county; plan on spending your first night here.

Get back on the Loyalist Parkway, also known as Highway 33, which will take you through Picton on your way east to Glenora. A ferry has crossed the Adolphus Reach at Glenora since the beginning of settlements by the United Empire Loyalists; yours is a free car-ferry operated by the province.

You'll arrive after a ten-minute trip at Adolphustown to begin a quiet 40 km stretch of road that clings to the water's edge as it passes 18th and 19th Century homesteads. As you reach Kingston, the lake is narrowing to become the source of the St. Lawrence River, one of the great rivers of the world, stretching for more than 1200 kilometers as it drains the world's largest fresh water source, the Great Lakes.

As you get into Kingston, look for Sir John A MacDonald Blvd. Take it south to the end, which is King Street. Turn left (east) on King. You'll be staring at Kingston Penitentiary and driving along the lake past Queen's University, through the historic neighbourhood of Sydenham Ward, past St. George's Cathedral and Kingston City Hall. The Thousand Islands extend from Wolfe Island, which you will see across the harbour from Kingston, to the narrows at Brockville. Don't visit Wolfe Island yet; you will cross it from the other side on your way home.

Continuing on you will cross the causeway across the Cataraqui River on up the hill to Fort Henry. A walk around Fort Henry provides spectacular views of Kinston to the right and the Thousand Islands to the left.

The St. Lawrence was discovered by Jacques Cartier in 1535. The early explorers used the St. Lawrence River as a highway to the interior of the continent. The Thousand Islands actually number 1,865. Some are just a few rocks sticking out of the water, while others are very large, like Wolfe Island, which is about 40 km long by about 14 km wide. The islands were formed almost 12,000 years at the end of the last ice age and they form a connecting bridge between the

Canadian Shield to the north and the Adirondack mountains to the south, in New York State. Geologically speaking, the connection is the Frontenac Arch; the narrow granite spur that bisects the region and provides the rugged character of the Thousand Islands. The narrow channel here provides a corridor for wildlife movement.

The boundary agreement in 1793 between the U.S. and Canada decided that no island would be split in two and that the boundary should be 100 yards from any shore. If that was not possible, the line would run right down the middle between the two shores. This explains why the U.S. / Canada boundary follows a zigzag line. Two-thirds of the Islands are in Canadian territory but the total acreage of the Canadian and American Islands is roughly equal.

It's is a nice drive down the Thousand Islands Parkway. When you leave Kingston, just keep to Highway 2; don't go back up to the 401. You will pass through Ganagoque and join the parkway heading toward Rockport; a good place for a stop and perhaps a boat cruise through the choicest part of the islands. You can continue as you please to Brockville or turn back to the 1000 Islands Bridge.

It is actually a series of bridges from island to island that was built in 1938, with Prime Minister William Mackenzie King and President Franklin Roosevelt in office. Over a distance of nearly 14 km, it takes you to New York State. Did I mention that you should bring your passport or other official identification to allow your brief visit to the States?

Clayton, New York sits on a peninsula surrounded by the St. Lawrence and is my favourite town on the American side. It was at its peak a century ago when the 1000 Islands were the playground of the rich. As many as 30 trains a day arrived from New York City to bring the summer visitors. During this period, many opulent homes and mansions were built in the area. The most famous was Boldt Castle, built by Mr. George C. Boldt, the owner of the Waldorf Astoria Hotel. Clayton is the home of the world famous Antique Boat Museum, the world's largest fresh water yacht and race boat museum. It is superb; if you love mahogany, don't miss it.

Carry on now eastward on your way to Cape Vincent, New York. Here you will find a privately operated 12-car ferry that will carry you across to the southern shore of Wolfe Island and back to Canada. Wolfe Island is a beautiful spot of farms and riverside views. Say hello to Don Cherry if you see him on his way to his cottage there. On the north side of the island is the Ontario government's free ferry, the Wolfe Islander III. It carries 55 cars per 20 minute trip to downtown Kingston. From there back home by the route of your choice.

CHAPTER 9
DRIVE ON!

Cars today are infinitely better in every respect than when the Boomers learned to drive. The safety technology packed into the latest cars – even the cheap ones – is sensational. The fuel economy, combined with near-zero emissions is an engineering marvel.

If we stay in shape us Boomers can continue to be the greatest car-loving generation of all time and the largest group of customers for the auto industry.

We ran to get our licenses the first day we could, but fewer and fewer teenagers today want to drive these great new cars. In fact, even 20-year-olds and 30-year-olds don't want to drive them. It's too expensive and too much hassle. The world has turned upside-down.

And it's not only in North America. In the U.K., the percentage of 17 to 20-year-olds with driving licenses fell from 48% in the early 1990s to 35% twenty years later.

Getting a driver's License? Now it's like taking a university course and nearly as expensive. And even a used car needs safety checks and emissions checks galore. Gas? $100 fill-up. Insurance? A few thousand dollars.

For at least the last twenty years, young people have sadly missed the fun and freedom of the affordable driving experience. Traffic is awful, parking is impossible, and everywhere they look there's some ambulance-chasing lawyer promising to sue the hell out of anyone involved in the slightest fender-bender.

No wonder Gen Y and the Millennials have retreated to the security of their smart phones and social media and have grown up as car-haters. They have avoided cars because it has become far too expensive and many believe they have better things to do with their time.

Here's a typically sour blogger on the subject:

If you have to pay an arm and a leg to own a car, get stuck in traffic, circle for 20 minutes to find a parking spot, and thus become frustrated and stressed – then it is not worth it.

Faster and more convenient to walk, bike, or take the subway or express buses with dedicated lanes where you don't get stuck.

That's the real problem with car ownership - you simply can't have millions of them in a limited urbanized area without running into these congestion and cost issues.

The projected social status and show-off thing will always come into play -- that is nothing new.

But in the end, what it all comes down to is being able to move around cheaply, conveniently and comfortably, and that equation has tilted away from the cult of the car.

Maybe we did join the cult of the car – but I loved it and won't apologize for it. I'm certainly glad that the quality of cars has improved so much and that they are far less harmful to the environment and I plan to continue enjoying the independence and freedom that cars provide long into the future.

Having said that I think I'll go back and watch that "23 ½ Hours" video again. Staying healthy is the real Job One.

And don't hesitate getting checked out in a Functional Driving Assessment now before you have to. You'll get excellent feedback which will improve your driving skills but also the peace of mind that you still have what it takes to continue to drive safely.

As soon as I finish this page I hit the send button to fire the whole thing off to the publisher. Tomorrow morning I'm off on another great road trip. Over to Montreal for a couple of days then along the North shore of the St. Lawrence River to Baie Comeau, across the Gulf of St. Lawrence by ferry to Matane for a drive around the Gaspe peninsula. Then on along the New Brunswick shore to Nova Scotia and turn north to Cape Breton. I'll do the circuit on the Cabot Trail and stop to visit the Alexander Graham Bell Historic Site at Baddeck.

Returning to New Brunswick I'll drive south along the Bay of Fundy, through Saint John and cross the border into Maine. I'll drive briefly back into Canada to visit FDR's Campobello then down the Maine. In southern New Hampshire I can pick up the I495 which takes me to the Mass Pike and then it's straight home (in about ten hours).

It's late May, the weather *should* be alright and I'm well ahead of the high traffic summer tourist season. the scenery will be great, and there will be a lot of amazing roads and historic sites. Cars really are freedom machines.

I hope you've enjoyed the book and have picked up a few things that will help you maintain yourself as a safe, licensed driver for the long term. Driving is a privilege and we all have to earn it in order to keep the roads as safe as possible. I accept that fact and will do my utmost to maintain my health and driving skills to continue on the open road for decades to come. I hope I see you out there with me.

ABOUT THE AUTHOR

Michael Vaughan is an automotive columnist, television host and successful businessman. He was host of Michael Vaughan Live and The Bottom Line on BNN for several years. Earlier in his career he was with CBC National as a reporter in Toronto, Halifax and the Ottawa Press Gallery. He likes nothing better than a good road trip and has driven widely on six continents.

Printed in Canada